WHEN EXPERIMENTS
TRAVEL

WHEN EXPERIMENTS
TRAVEL

CLINICAL TRIALS *and the* GLOBAL SEARCH
FOR HUMAN SUBJECTS

ADRIANA PETRYNA

PRINCETON UNIVERSITY PRESS

PRINCETON AND OXFORD

Copyright © 2009 by Princeton University Press

Published by Princeton University Press, 41 William Street, Princeton, New Jersey 08540
In the United Kingdom: Princeton University Press, 6 Oxford Street, Woodstock,
Oxfordshire OX20 1TW

Library of Congress Cataloging-in-Publication Data

Petryna, Adriana, date.
When experiments travel : clinical trials and the global search for human subjects /
Adriana Petryna.
p. ; cm.
Includes bibliographical references and index.
ISBN 978-0-691-12656-2 (hardcover : alk. paper)—ISBN 978-0-691-12657-9 (pbk. : alk. paper)
1. Clinical trials—Moral and ethical aspects.   2. Drugs—Testing—Moral and ethical aspects.
I. Title.
[DNLM: 1. Clinical Trials as Topic.   2. Human Experimentation—ethics.   3. Drug Design.
4. Internationality.   5. Patient Selection.
QV 20.5 P498w 2009]
R853.C55P48 2009
610.72'4—dc22   2008040866

British Library Cataloging-in-Publication Data is available

This book has been composed in Minion with
ITC Franklin Gothic and Bauer Bodoni display

Printed on acid-free paper. ∞

press.princeton.edu

Printed in the United States of America

3   5   7   9   10   8   6   4   2

For João and Andre

CONTENTS

꒐◈꒑

ABBREVIATIONS

ACHRE	Advisory Committee on Human Radiation Experiments
ANVISA	Agência Nacional de Vigilância Sanitária (Brazilian National Health Surveillance Agency)
BMIS	Bioresearch Monitoring Information System File (FDA)
CONEP	Comissão Nacional de Ética em Pesquisa (Brazilian National Committee on Research Ethics)
CRO	contract research organization
EMEA	European Agency for the Evaluation of Medicinal Products
ERT	enzyme replacement therapy
FDA	U.S. Food and Drug Administration
FDAMA	Food and Drug Administration Modernization Act
GCP	Good Clinical Practice
GFHR	Global Forum for Health Research
HEW	U.S. Department of Health, Education and Welfare
HHS	U.S. Department of Health and Human Services
ICH	International Conference on Harmonisation of Technical Requirements for Registration of Pharmaceuticals for Human Use
ICMJE	International Committee of Medical Journal Editors
ICTRP	International Clinical Trials Registry Platform
IND	investigational new drug
IOWH	Institute for OneWorld Health
IRB	institutional review board
NDA	new drug application
NIH	U.S. National Institutes of Health
OHRP	Office for Human Research Protections (HHS)
OIG	Office of Inspector General (HHS)
PEPFAR	President's Emergency Plan for AIDS Relief
PIH	Partners In Health
PT	Partido dos Trabalhadores (Brazilian Workers Party)
R&D	research and development
RCT	randomized controlled trial
SAE	serious adverse events

SMO	site management organization
SUS	Sistema Único de Saúde (Brazilian national health system)
TRIPS	trade-related aspects of intellectual property rights
WHO	World Health Organization
WTO	World Trade Organization

WHEN EXPERIMENTS
TRAVEL

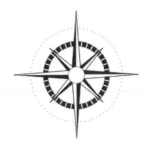

EXPERIMENTAL FIELDS

The Search for Human Subjects

If I drive two miles down the road that takes me to the supermarkets and re-
tail shops of the midwestern town where I grew up, I will pass the local
branch of Across-the-Globe-Research (AGR). A freestanding office space,
newly built, with a redbrick exterior and white casement windows, the
building is surrounded by a parking lot. The AGR facility looks like a standard suburban medical practice, but it is not quite that. It is an investigative
research site that conducts clinical trials for the pharmaceutical industry.
Clinical trials are studies designed to systematically evaluate new drugs or
new ways of using known treatments in humans. They are a way to meet the
requirement that the safety and effectiveness of drugs or treatments be established before they enter the market. Yet trials are imperfect and, at times,
biased instruments that may or may not yield the most complete evidence
about a drug's benefits and risks.

Inside AGR, one spring day in 2005, a bedraggled patient-volunteer, accompanied by an escort who appeared to be his caregiver, sat waiting for his
name to be called by a physician who was standing behind a glass pane—
much like a bank teller, I thought. The physician asked the patient whether
he had experienced any side effects from taking an experimental drug. The
answer was no, and the doctor passed him a new dose. The patient left. He
would return regularly over a prescribed period. According to the research
protocol, some visits were brief, like this one. Others involved more detailed

physical observations to gather data related to the clinical trial's specific objectives.[1]

AGR's physician-employees are specialists in neurology, gastroenterology, endocrinology, and psychiatry. They enroll volunteers from a pool of new patients in their private practices and from AGR's own, and larger, patient database. Regardless of the source of the trial participants, though, AGR, as the investigative site, bears ultimate responsibility for compliance with regulations governing human subjects research.

The window separating the doctor from the patient-volunteer was a cold reminder of a loss of intimacy in medical care—a loss that social scientists have lamented as moral codes guiding physician behavior are increasingly defined by nonmedical outsiders, lawyers, for example.[2] Physicians at this facility preferred to be distant. According to AGR's business manager, whom I will call Evan (and whom I spoke to that afternoon), most physicians here feel that research practice interferes with their regular clinical practice. They would rather not mix them. The benefits of this arrangement apparently outweighed the conflicts of interest that might have been built into it: "When experimental drugs are available, of course, physicians feel compelled to enroll their patients." The transactions at this site and Evan's confident statements speak to the distinctive public presence of clinical trials and to the shifting boundaries between medical research and medical care.

Global pharmaceutical sales reached $712 billion in 2007.[3] North America accounts for almost half of total sales, and there is an accelerated growth in the new markets of Latin America, Asia, and Eastern Europe.[4] Today, more than 70 percent of all medical visits in the United States result in at least one "drug mention," a term used to denote the prescription, continuation, or provision of a drug. On average, two drug mentions are recorded per medical visit.[5] Antidepressants are the most highly prescribed drugs, followed by medications to combat high blood pressure, anticholesterol agents, antiarthritics, and antiasthmatics. This phenomenal pharmaceutical expansion has been coupled with an unprecedented surge in the number of health professionals and patients recruited into clinical research in the United States and in middle- and low-income countries. In recent decades, access to experimental therapies has broadened, particularly in the areas of AIDS, cancer, and genetic treatments, and ambitious federal and industry efforts are under way to recruit more people for clinical trials in the United States and abroad.

Different kinds of patients have different stakes in clinical trials. As trial participation becomes a form of mainstream medicine, the desperately ill might accept clinical trials as their best medical option rather than as "mere" experimentation. For many, taking part in a trial means getting access to better medical monitoring than what is routinely provided in industrialized medicine. For those with no health insurance, trials are sometimes the only pathway to needed treatment. And for people who do not have stable jobs, drug trials and other kinds of trials might be a source of income.[6]

Precise figures of the number of trial participants and clinical trials carried out in the United States, let alone worldwide, are hard to come by. This is in part because the Food and Drug Administration (FDA), the principal agency regulating drugs, medical devices, and biological products used by Americans, is unable to identify all ongoing clinical trials and their associated trial sites (OIG 2007). As of 2008, 65,755 trials sponsored by federal agencies and private industry were listed on ClinicalTrials.gov, a service of the U.S. National Institutes of Health designed to provide up-to-date information for those interested in locating clinical trials. It is estimated that each year, more than 2.3 million people participate in clinical trials in the United States alone. Between 2000 and 2005, the FDA audited fewer than 1 percent of the 350,000 trials sites that the Office of Inspector General has estimated are active worldwide (ibid.:19).

The truth is that governmental agencies have little control over this experimental field, and as a general public we know little about the design of research protocols, the conditions under which trials are carried out, or the dependability of the evidence about a drug's benefits and risks. As recent withdrawals of drugs from the market illustrate, experimentation extends beyond the duration of the clinical trial—with potentially deleterious effects. For example, approximately 6 million American women were using hormone replacement therapy when, in 2002, the Women's Health Initiative discovered that the potential harms, including increased risks of breast cancer, heart disease, stroke, and blood clots, outweighed the benefits of the treatment. Similarly, physicians had prescribed a popular nonsteroidal anti-inflammatory drug to 84 million people before the drug was removed from the market in 2004, after evidence of cardiovascular risk came to light.

Today, the majority of clinical research endeavors are industry sponsored. In 1980, industry funded 32 percent of clinical research. By 2000, the figure had soared to 62 percent. AGR began business in the mid-1990s and has been expanding ever since. It has a dozen affiliated research sites, located in diverse socioeconomic enclaves and towns in the United States and in Eastern Europe and Eurasia that run all phases of clinical trials. One midwestern U.S. site is operated by a Polish-born psychiatrist with a busy adult practice. This doctor works in three area hospitals and supervises trials involving a largely Eastern European immigrant population. The site advertises its staff as being multilingual. Another site is located in a psychiatric counseling center in the heart of a once-prosperous coal-mining town. This facility is also run by a psychiatrist who has a private practice and is employed by local hospitals. Another of AGR's sites is located at the southeastern shore, near large retirement communities. After Hurricane Katrina, the Gulf Coast site stopped enrolling research subjects.

Evan, my AGR contact, is an articulate and hardworking fifty-year-old businessman. When we met that day at his office, he looked fit and was casually dressed in a worn, light-blue oxford shirt with the sleeves rolled up. Evan also facilitated overseas drug testing, and he explained the draw of carrying out drug studies in Eastern Europe and Eurasia. Subjects there are apt to be accommodating, he said. They receive Western medical treatments they otherwise could not pay for, and they adhere to trial procedures and do what is asked of them. Physicians in those regions are known to be competent, but poorly paid; they gravitate toward the money research brings. According to Evan, they are willing to become study monitors, providing support for other physician-investigators and making sure that research protocols are properly executed. That task pays considerably more than what a Russian physician earns for treating patients, Evan told me.

This expert seemed to move effortlessly between the business of clinical trials overseas and that in the United States. Fifty miles west of AGR, in a nearby state, are the headquarters of several contract research organizations (CROs), including two former employers of Evan. Unlike AGR, a small company that focuses solely on running trials, CROs offer a wider set of services to pharmaceutical, biotechnology, and medical-device companies. They organize and monitor all stages of global multisited trials and guide clients through complex national regulatory environments. In his previous capacity as a leader of business development for a CRO, Evan told me, he had gained "a good sense of how the international marketplace for clinical testing works." He said he had also acquired regulatory and legal knowledge there and developed networks of contacts in the United States and abroad that came in handy when he created his own company. In 2003, AGR investors approached him. As he recalls, "They said, 'We want you to work this company from a business development perspective, and we'll give you a piece of it all.'" His statement suggests that in clinical research, the chain of entrepreneurial stakeholders is getting longer and more decentralized, rather than becoming streamlined.

Monitoring rooms, laboratory space, and storage make up this local AGR office. Researchers can conduct more specialized trial-related assessments and tests within a mile of the office, at private medical facilities. AGR investigators are also attending physicians in the acute care and outpatient services of nearby hospitals, and AGR collaborates with other physicians in the region, who refer patients to this investigative site. According to Evan, AGR is overwhelmed with industry contracts. Pharmaceutical sponsors need study subjects, and, as he put it, "We can't take in patients fast enough." Demand overtakes supply, in part, because the U.S. landscape of commercial clinical research "suffers from dire shortages of investigator sites and patients," in Evan's words. Starting in the early nineties, clinical research in the United States began moving out of academic medical settings, where it had been principally conducted, to local hospitals and primary-care settings and private investigative sites such as AGR. Evan is part of a growing group of subcontracted professionals who make up the so-called clinical trials industry that facilitates a decisive step in the global science of drug development. He marshals qualified investigators and patients, and his company piggybacks drug testing onto existing health care infrastructures. His work is part of a thriving and expanding global experimental enterprise, one whose scope and broader implications are largely unknown.

Anthropology and the Global Clinical Trial

The pharmaceutical industry is the major producer of today's therapeutic armamentarium, and it is increasingly outsourcing and offshoring clinical research. This book is about the business of clinical trials.[7] It examines the organizational cultures of industry-sponsored clinical research, probing scientific, ethical, and regulatory practices. The book traces the worldwide expansion of this experimental enterprise, and it explores how it is integrated into medicine and public health in both rich and poor settings. I began investigating clinical research (mainly related to chronic diseases and to new genetic therapies) in 2001 and continued, charting its movement to Eastern Europe and Latin America, for the next several years. The entrepreneurial world of clinical trials is composed of contract research organizations; patient recruitment firms; for-profit research ethics review boards; and stand-alone investigative research sites that are nestled in urban and suburban communities in the United States and around the world. The clinical trials industry accounts for roughly one-third of all clinical development expenditures. While the pharmaceutical industry's revenue growth has leveled off somewhat, the clinical trials industry has boomed. What, precisely, is the relation between the drug industry's stagnation and the clinical trials industry's rise?[8]

I initially focused my study on how the clinical trials industry evolved and has been operating in the United States. I paid particular attention to the work of contract research organizations, the biggest and most profitable sector of this industry. Speaking with corporate executives, administrators, and scientists, I asked them how they defined their work and overcame operational and technical problems, and how they navigated ethical guidelines, national regulations, and business practices. Because one of my chief concerns was the question of scientific integrity, I then charted the evidence-making practices that have evolved with the offshoring of clinical trials (to Poland, for example). I engaged trial managers and monitors, along with publicly funded academic scientists and national health authorities, and I also considered the effects of privately funded clinical research in ailing public health systems (in Brazil, for example).

In my inquiry, I saw the promises and perils of the global clinical trial taking form, and in this book I distill the fundamentals of what I learned from the many parties involved. A few caveats are in order. I am not a bioscientist, and my purpose here is not to evaluate the pharmacological or clinical science entailed in drug development. As an anthropologist, I have written about the social and political implications of science and technology in the context of nuclear disaster and global pharmaceuticals.[9] Much has been written about the social construction of the evidentiary process in clinical trials—how the evidence-making process is itself laden with financial conflicts of interest.[10] Not much has been said about the practical and technical concerns that surround current strategies of clinical research and how they affect collective and public health processes downstream. My study focuses on these latter issues, and I am committed to bringing anthropological knowledge to bear on ethics and policy debates. But it is ultimately the work of scientists, doctors, and regulators to appraise the safety and efficacy of new therapies. This book is not "antiscience," nor is it intended to undercut the social value of the research enterprise. Pharmaceutical innovation contributes critically to the alleviation of the global burden of disease. As I address the changing precepts governing clinical trials and how experimental groups are identified and constituted, I ask: what value systems bring researchers, physicians, and patients into trials? More broadly, if clinical research increasingly serves as a surrogate to underfunded state health-care systems, how do we assess drug value, minimize investments in drugs that are either unsafe or marginally beneficial, and maximize institutional investments in global access to the drugs that are both safe and beneficial? Throughout the book, I give voice to the perspectives of national regulators, industry figures, and their critics. How do they see the dimensionality of the problem and the implications of their work in terms of control over methods, researchers, subjects, and ethical issues? In shedding light on actual practices and decision-making processes, my goal is to foster less partisan and more comprehensive understandings of the human dimensions of scientific innovation. I believe that it is the task of social science to produce nuanced and people-centered forms of knowledge, correcting asymmetries of information and helping to promote, to the best of our ability, informed consent, human protection, and safety in medical and research settings.

In chapter 1, I present some of the book's main actors and juxtapose their knowledge bases and practices. I highlight the main factors underlying the growth of the clinical trials industry and offshoring of clinical trials. What is taking place is experimentality and not just fine-tuned, randomized controlled trials that people are free to choose whether or not to enter into. I discuss controversies that have recently framed debates over globalizing clinical research and interpret them from a strategic industry standpoint. While trials of AZT treatment using placebos in Africa and elsewhere may be limit cases, such trials permit us to explore the gaps between international ethical guidelines and the social and political realities of research. In zones of crisis, protection and safety considerations are weighed against immediate health benefits or the knowledge to be gained, leading to a cost-effective variability in ethical standards. As health risk becomes a resource for capital, ethical variability becomes a core value and a presumed modus operandi in globalized clinical research. What work is to be done to guarantee accountability and to link experimental biologies to regimes of protection?

The clinical trials industry is a crucial, highly mobile and profitable arm of the pharmaceutical industry; it is both domestic and international in scope. Chapter 2 explores the outsourcing and offshoring of clinical trials, past and present, and how they interconnect with the dynamics of drug development and regulation in the United States. Experimentality as an instrumental use of humans in research was, arguably, already present at the outset of modern drug regulation (Marks 1997). I show how a risk-benefit approach to different research contexts evolved and is being applied in global settings. I also elaborate on the problems and limits of this instrumental use of humans, as well as tease out the logic, loopholes, and gaps in existing regulatory structures that legitimate it internationally. The scientists I knew were troubled about safety problems being detected only after the fact. They articulate surprising connections between this failure to detect and trial offshoring.

Uncertainties have plagued the research enterprise at home, but what happens when experiments travel? In chapter 3, I take the reader to Eastern Europe, where I investigated the organization and spatial mobility of offshored trials and probed the limits of oversight and accountability (understood as the ability to track clinical trials, maintain scientific integrity, or reduce research-related risk). What are the institutional arrangements allowing experimentality to rise and (sooner or later) fall? Why is it that public debates over commodified patients and expertise seldom arise? How to reconcile images of free movement and riskless profit with the actual forms of risk and liability on the ground? The quotidian operations generating efficacy and safety data become ethnographic contexts from which one can observe the benefits and risks of private-sector science as it is rapidly integrated into public health systems and emerging drug markets.

Once clinical trials data have been sent off to corporate headquarters, new medical fields emerge locally. In chapter 4, I turn to Brazil and investigate the aftermath of clinical trials. It is in this posttrial stage that issues such as continuity of treatment and ongoing control of data by sponsors—sometimes not anticipated in contracts or informed consent forms—must be addressed. Posttrial subjects-turned-patients and -consumers continue to need medicines that are now on the market yet out of their financial reach. Meanwhile, trial sponsors continue to exert control over study data in the drug-marketing phase. Throughout the chapter, I show how academic scientists are dealing with the overwhelming demand made by patients and marketers on doctors to prescribe, and on the state to provide, new high-cost medicines whose benefits are not unequivocally established. As they dissect the comparative value of new drugs, these Brazilian scientists convey a systemic knowledge of the political economy of pharmaceuticals and the inequities that it can generate locally. They are creating alternative treatment protocols in dialogue with international experts and in partnership with national health policy makers. Their story is not about an evidence-based scientific orthodoxy. It is about how local actors, states, and patients in a low-income setting create institutions to address at times appalling disparities between drug value and price and the complex political and market factors that impede their efforts.

It is also about new collaborations and experiments that aim to make needed medicines accessible and their provision sustainable.

Whether they work directly for the clinical trials industry as scientists and monitors, are occasionally recruited as paid investigators, or remain outsider-critics, my interlocutors in the United States, Brazil, and Poland cite challenges and risks that, despite the oversight of regulatory and ethics review boards, are being produced in the global economy of research. In their efforts to improve scientific integrity, reduce risk, or negotiate drug costs, they illuminate situations that are not unique to their respective countries. In the concluding chapter, I draw these various threads and experiences together—scientific, commercial, public—in a discussion of medical innovation in global public health.

Clinical trials are part of charged social and political landscapes that link diverse participants—researchers, trial subjects, health professionals, corporate executives, regulators, policy makers, patient-consumers, and shareholders—to a host of calculable and incalculable hopes, benefits, profits, and risks. Experimentality, now an explicitly global phenomenon, enfolds public and private actors and interests into interconnected data-producing sites. It also provokes questions about how exactly the boundaries between research and practice are negotiated in various health settings. *When Experiments Travel* identifies elements of this multifaceted enterprise and weaves them into a global ethnography. Seen from this perspective, ideas of the therapeutic are more than scientifically or statistically determined constructs. They are also concepts of value, deeply embedded in economic, political, and technological imperatives. This book brings into view some of the convoluted contexts of the production of clinical trial data. In so doing, it excavates sources of knowledge that can help us rethink the criteria with which we define medical progress and, in the process, redirect our political commitments and investments.

CHAPTER ONE

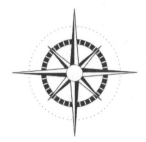

ETHICAL VARIABILITY

Why Are Clinical Trials Globalizing?

In the view of Dr. Lee, a company scientist who coordinates clinical trials in Eastern Europe, public distrust of the clinical trials process is rampant in the United States and in Western Europe, and "it is becoming a major barrier to our work." For him, the growth of clinical research offshore expresses a straightforward yet unsettling value system: "If a doctor or nurse asked you if you were willing to put a family member in a clinical trial, and if it was not a life-or-death issue, would you do it? The answer would most likely be no. The fact is that all of us, drug researchers and consumers, are economically dependent on other people's willingness to say yes." This expert knows that landscapes of experimentation evolve in a kind of give-and-take where people with unmet medical needs are willing to say yes to the movement of global capital and scientific and medical commodities.

Consider Poland. The country had one of the highest rates of cardiovascular-disease-related deaths in the world, and it has recently developed impressive preventive apparatuses to reverse this trend. Poland's leading heart institutes and public hospitals have become preferred destinations for trials of therapies ranging from hypertension treatments to invasive surgical procedures. Hospital administrators so welcomed these trials that by the late 1990s a prestigious cardiology institute in Warsaw was "awash in thrombolytics," or clot-busting drugs, according to one businessman and former physician coordinating trials in Poland. He suggested to me in 2005 that clinical trials were a social good, an integral part of health-care delivery. "Not a single ampule in the institute was purchased. Each patient who needed treatment got it from a clinical trial."[1] Here underserved patients are experimental subjects whose added value lies in the fact that they have not previously been treated with the particular drug or class of drugs under study. As a clinical research expert told me, untreated patients of this sort minimize the chance of specific drug-drug interactions and "offer a more likely prospect of minimizing the number of variables affecting results and a better chance of showing drug effectiveness." That people in lower-income countries (just like people in affluent ones) might be consuming several drugs or self-medicating, often unsystematically, has not deterred companies from pursuing particular sites in which they imagine the "naive" (i.e., those who have not been diagnosed or treated for the condition under study) might be found—in a poorer region or hospital, for example.[2]

Certainly, the human research enterprise is about obtaining valuable data that can get drugs approved. But it is also about creating new experimental infrastructures, remediating old ones, and expanding market frontiers.[3] "Pharmaceuticals are the new gold," as Dr. Paulo Picon, a southern Brazilian cardiologist and public health expert, told me skeptically. He is a staunch critic of the increasing use of clinical trials as a means of introducing high-cost medicines in Brazil's ailing public health-care system. "After a trial ends, the industry enlists doctors to prescribe and patients to demand drugs from the state." Pharmaceutical costs overburden the system, and "often these new drugs have not even been approved here and their benefits are not yet clearly established."

Whether they work in the United States, Poland, or Brazil, my informants raise crucial issues that go to the heart of the globalized clinical trial. Are clinical trials exploitative or are they social goods or some combination of both? How are research protocols designed and data produced? How do the results of clinical trials strengthen or undermine the delivery of affordable and effective interventions? Who is ultimately responsible for the experimental subject's immediate and long-term well-being?

Pharmaceutical research and development (R&D) includes laboratory and animal studies and clinical testing in humans—in the United States both are subject to federal regulation.[4] R&D spending has soared over the past three decades, from $1.1 billion in 1975 to $44.5 billion in 2007. For the top ten pharmaceutical firms—more than half of which are based in the United States—approximately 40 percent of this amount is spent on clinical trials.[5] Clinical trials involving new drugs are generally divided into four phases. In Phase 1 trials, researchers determine the safety and safe dose range of experimental drugs and detect their toxicological side effects in a small group (20–80) of healthy volunteers. In Phase 2 trials, 100 to 300 people are recruited for assessment of the drug's efficacy and further evaluation of its safety. In Phase 3 trials, investigators administer the study drug to larger groups (1,000–3,000) of people to confirm its effectiveness, scrutinize side effects, compare it to other treatments, and collect information on optimal use. These trials are frequently coordinated across multiple centers, which, increasingly, are located worldwide. Phase 4 trials, also known as postmarketing surveillance, are primarily observational and nonexperimental studies in which companies and regulators collate data on the drug's risks and benefits once it enters the market. Postmarketing surveillance involves millions of people but in practice remains vastly underdeveloped.[6]

In 2000, representatives from diverse interest groups met to reflect on the state of clinical research in the United States, which, they said, was contributing to an overall decline in drug innovation. They agreed that, in spite of greater research funding from the National Institutes of Health (NIH) and revolutions in basic biomedical science, clinical research is "increasingly encumbered by high costs, slow results, lack of funding, regulatory burdens, fragmented infrastructure, incompatible databases, and a shortage of qualified investigators and willing participants" (Sung et al. 2003:1278). Moreover, the U.S. clinical research environment limits the translation of basic scientific concepts into human studies and medical practice. The environment must be improved, and the president and U.S. Congress must enact bold new approaches. If not, they claimed, the "data and information produced by the basic science enterprise will not result in a tangible public benefit" (ibid.:1279; see also Rosenberg 2003).[7]

The clinical trials industry promises to address and overcome such technical and regulatory barriers. Since the 1980s, pharmaceutical companies have increasingly outsourced clinical research.[8] As the CEO of one contract research organization told me, "About 60 percent of all clinical development costs are spent on Phase 2 and Phase 3 trials. So the big money is there." He stated that drug firms outsource "about half of their initial toxicological or Phase 1 studies," and that CROs like his are also engaged in postapproval marketing studies to promote new products. The CRO market size is estimated at $10 billion and growing. Hundreds of CROs operate worldwide, employing nearly one hundred thousand professionals who implement clinical trials protocols for the pharmaceutical industry.[9]

The geography of clinical testing is changing dramatically. In 2005, 40 percent of all trials were carried out in emerging markets, up from 10 percent in 1991 (Lustgarden 2005:68). Figures are available for some firms. GlaxoSmithKline ran 29 percent of its trials outside the United States and Western Europe in 2004; by 2007, that figure grew to 50 percent. Wyeth Pharmaceuticals conducted half of its trials outside the United States in 2004; that figure rose to 70 percent in 2006. Merck conducted half of its clinical trials outside the United States in 2004, an increase of 45 percent since 1999 (Schmit 2005). According to recent industry statistics, Central-Eastern Europe has the highest volume of patients (6.27) enrolled per investigative site, followed by the Asia-Pacific region (5.78), South-Central America (4.56), Western Europe (3.08), and the United States (1.92) (Parexel 2008: 135). Between 1995 and 2006, the highest annual growth in active investigators occurred in Russia, Argentina, India, Poland, Brazil, and China. Of these select countries, as of 2006, Russia had the highest number of investigators enrolled with the FDA (623), followed by India (464), Argentina (462), Poland (322), China (307), and Brazil (292).[10]

As the clinical trials enterprise becomes ever more outsourced and offshored, it also becomes increasingly decentralized and more difficult to track. While we have estimates of numbers of investigators involved, estimates for the number of clinical trials actually being initiated worldwide vary considerably. In March 2006, a member of a World Health Organization initiative to create a global registry of clinical trials told me, "Our best guess is that 20,000 new trials are initiated worldwide annually. But take this 'guesstimate' with a grain of salt." A global field of experimental activity is booming and experts struggle to simply keep count.[11]

Companies are free to move medical research to cost-effective sites around the globe. Meanwhile, the subjects of research depend upon local and national communities to mediate their participation in clinical trials and to protect them from harms that may be associated with such participation. An international trial registry could help us to better account for this corporate–human subjects disjuncture and to gauge the relevance of international ethical guidelines and capacities of local and national institutions to protect patient-citizens in an era of global experimentality.

🔸◇🔸

The decision regarding whether to carry out clinical trials, where, and how is as much a scientific as it is an economic and political one.[12] This political economy bears the stamp of a set of practices inherent in the pharmaceutical industry as it has evolved in North America in the twentieth century. Specifically, I have in mind the history of research among minorities and so-called cooperative patients and professional guinea pigs. I also have in mind the power the industry exerts over evidence making and drug regulatory policy.[13] Some of these operations are empirically accessible, while others are proprietary and part of the pharmaceutical black box. The anthropological challenge is to engage the transparent and public ways in which private-sector research undergoes global restructuring today.[14]

Anthropologist Carol Greenhouse urges those studying "closed institutions" to move beyond an analytics of "hidden transcripts" and to chart transcripts "that surface in plain sight" (2005:364). In her analysis of legal responses to the 9/11 tragedy, particularly the establishment of closed military tribunals, Greenhouse focuses on what she calls the "visible junctures" and "discursive trails" of state and legal institutions—less emphasis on the elusive black box and more attention on the sites where the demands for "invisibility and visibility confront each other" (Sivaramakrishnan 2005: 326). In this way, the anthropologist finds the means of objectifying "emergent lines of political restructuring," and thus interpreting them and, hopefully, identifying alternative possibilities of action.

In this book, I take the operations of the clinical trials industry as a window into global drug development and the ways experimental subjects and therapeutic evidence are constituted. I collected the professional histories of leading scientists and entrepreneurs who founded the industry in the 1970s and 1980s. In doing so, I produced a recent history of outsourced clinical research, tracing it back to the postwar boom in pharmaceutical production and to regulatory and health-care system changes in the United States.

In 2001, I began to engage U.S.-based contract researchers and clinical trials professionals—scientists, former physicians, M.D./Ph.D.'s, business-people and marketers—who spoke openly and plainly about all aspects, both good and bad, of the science of drug development. In reflecting on their craft, they gave me deeper insights into recent media coverage of the hazards of drugs and how they might have been created. Executives also allowed me to follow the activities of some of their affiliates overseas. The men and women I spoke with saw themselves as innovators operating at the productive margins of very large and powerful institutions—academia and multinational pharmaceutical companies—for which many of them had previously worked. In their self-presentation, these professionals objected to the occasional media vilification of their work as a corruption of the scientific method and a breach of ethics.[15] They are largely drawn from the same labor pool as pharmaceutical and biotech employees, but questions are periodically raised about their "degree of independence from their pharmaceutical-industry clients" (Shuchman 2007:1365). The industry's main trade group suggests that the scrutiny is misplaced, as "[s]ponsors call the shots. Sponsors shoulder final responsibility for the trials they design" (ClinPage 2007). One CRO professional told me that sponsors exhibit an unrealistic "bravado" in their demands, and that he and his colleagues were engaged in a "less delusional" form of work. He believed that most pharmaceutical clients were largely "out of touch" with the realities and exigencies of on-the-ground research.

These physicians and scientists, "purely operational," on the one hand, were also troubleshooters and fastidious with detail. They conveyed a heightened sense of the risks of the competitive world they labored in, of its responsibilities, rules, and penalties. They deployed informal moralities and sometimes had to choose between alternatives that were not obviously right or wrong. In this sense, my anthropological work differs from that of a journalist; it is not exposé-oriented and I do not have the entry points to undertake such work. Rather, these subcontracted actors offer a crash course on the integrity and weaknesses of global expert systems, forms of science, capitalism, and law—and in how these translate into social practices that can be considered, contested, or debated. In taking them on their own terms, I ask: What ethical deliberations and actions are possible in arenas fraught with high financial and political stakes? What is transparency and what are the risks of distortion? How are those risks distributed, deferred, or mitigated, and what spaces of negotiation open in their wake?

Their critiques, however, should not be taken at face value; they must be understood in the context of a mutable research ecology that is fraught with competition. Two executives from another company referred to their business sector as an "opportunistic" by-product of "an overinflated industry" that needed to be "downsized."

When I asked a researcher about risks in drug testing, he expressed frustration with the clinical trials operational model, specifically with regard to "how dumb the drug-testing process is with respect to detecting harms." Trial sponsors exercise significant control over the definition of a reportable adverse event; it seemed that exercising critical independence allowed him and his colleagues to identify new areas of expertise and needs in drug development that would, in turn, lead to the expansion of their outsourced enterprise. After 2004, and in the wake of the FDA's issuance of safety warnings for several approved drugs, this scientist's company (like others) attempted to differentiate itself from competitors by promoting its own drug safety–enhancing niche, promoting technological strategies aimed at lowering risk and improving the "robustness" (i.e., reliability) of scientific results.

Contract research organizations are thriving businesses at home and abroad. As a former CEO, whom I will call Rob, told me during a conversation in 2004, "There has been a big evolution from the 1980s until now, from simple capabilities to our being able to run entire global programs. By the mid-1990s, companies like ours were planting flags all over the globe." Members of this subcontracted community gave me insights, drawn from their own experiences, into cultures of drug development and the technical and political challenges they face. As they invent the means to make drugs approvable and marketable, they claim to be the creators of a "translational science" in their own right. By and large, they stressed lawfulness and technical competence. Their narratives also conformed to business models, and as such they were strategies for creating value. Juxtaposing what these actors told me with the accounts of other actors in the clinical trials "food chain" helped me see the remedial kind of work the clinical trials industry, and specifically CROs, perform. The professionals' narratives attest to concrete problems and unknowns that are only partially addressed and temporarily fixed.

CROs put a premium on time and speed. They assess the regulatory environments of prospective countries in at least two ways: on the basis of "country approval time" and "country activation time." The first term refers to the time it takes for companies to obtain approval to begin a clinical trial in a particular country. This is dependent on factors related to internal government bureaucracy, the quality of national and local ethics committees and inspection regimes, and procedures and authorizations involved in drug importing. The second term refers to the time it takes for a company to get a study up and running. This involves finding centers of research excellence, training personnel, recruiting patients, and shipping experimental compounds to the sites. Approval and activation times inform a fluid map of locations where, at any given moment, trials could be quickly launched that would result in high-quality clinical data. The same terms also identify countries that should be pursued further or invested in (as well as sites that should be avoided) and countries in which the drug under study could be marketed. Bureaucrats, evidence-gatherers, and moneymakers are all entangled in what one well-regarded industry consultant described to me as "cutthroat commodity work."

Given the emphasis on time, speed, and profitability, I am particularly concerned with how scientific integrity is maintained and ensured in new clinical trials frontiers, as well as with conveying the ethical reflections of the diverse actors involved. Clinical trials data must be gathered in an objective and dispassionate manner, but "given the high cost of drug development," as Rob told me, "we don't even go to the clinical trials stage unless we have evidence that a drug works." His main scientific adviser questioned the mechanics of this evidence-gathering process: "Companies can now pick and choose populations" to get the data they need, "in order to get a most pronounced drug benefit signal as well as a 'no-harm' signal." The risk-benefit ratio of various research settings is subject to economic constraints; the "scientific" rationale of protocols is often at cross-purposes with clinical realities and can introduce harms that, if present, would prove difficult to objectify after the fact.

To get an on-the-ground understanding of the offshoring of clinical trials, I carried out a comparative ethnographic inquiry in two popular trial destinations and emerging pharmaceutical markets: Poland and Brazil. In the pharmaceutical lexicon, both countries were seen as "pivotal," that is, they had the largest pharmaceutical market share for their regions and were vital to the industry's presence and expansion in their respective regions. Executives of two midsized CROs, which I will call Tem/po and AR/CH, allowed me to speak with the managers of their affiliates in Poland.[16] I carried out this study in 2005, when Poland had reached its peak in the globalized trial market. I spoke at length with executives, and they put me in contact with their subcontracted investigators and clinical trials monitors. I also interviewed some of the industry representatives as well as regulatory officers and lawyers with whom these firms' personnel interacted regularly (see chapter 3).

Each professional, occupying his/her specific role, repeatedly emphasized the productivity, seamlessness, and transparency of the whole enterprise. They were proud of the safe and competitive environment they had made. Much of their work entailed hiring and managing study monitors (also known as clinical research associates). These detail-oriented young professionals (holding medical or advanced scientific degrees) review trial records, ensure compliance with the protocol, and make sure data are "clean," that is, without evidence of protocol violation or fraud. An "excess of monitoring" is thought to guarantee the much sought-after scientific integrity and value of the data being produced (value in the sense that the data collected at a particular site would be usable in the context of a drug approval process). The monitors CROs employ literally protect the value of the data.[17] Yet the same monitoring that led to robust data was also a thin veil for an otherwise weak legal and medical infrastructure and, ultimately, masked a void in patient protection. In the memorable words of one of AR/CH's Eastern European managers, "We don't see patients, we see data." His country was in the midst of applying stricter regulations linked to its European Union (EU) membership, and the clinical trials industry, sensing longer "country approval time" and regulatory delays, was quickly moving into Russia and the Balkans.[18] I joined an AR/CH executive on one of his trips to Moscow, where his company had subcontracted with a local company supplying study monitors; his aim was to carry out surprise inspections on these monitors. As I conducted fieldwork in these outsourced worlds, it became apparent that their operations were far from airtight. It became more difficult to reconcile images of riskless profit in new clinical trials frontiers with the actual problems and liabilities that the local professionals I knew actually dealt with on the ground.

During the summers of 2003–2006, I worked in southern Brazil with industry-sponsored researchers and with physicians carrying out publicly sponsored research in a university hospital. Over the years, I also engaged academic scientists, policy makers, state prosecutors, and citizens as they were drawn into the contested field of access to high-cost medicines, particularly as it evolved in the aftermath of clinical trials (see chapter 4). In the early and mid-1990s, Brazil was *terra nova* for international clinical research, often used as a site for "rescue studies" (involving salvaging drugs that had failed in earlier clinical testing or while on the market). Like Poland, Brazil took a lead in embracing neoliberal reforms and opening new markets. The country had wholeheartedly embraced global trade rules, and industrialists now boasted that the country's clinical trials market was one of the fastest growing in the world.

A senior research scientist for a large pharmaceutical firm operating in Brazil confidently told me, "No one pays better attention to the ethical guidelines than we do." However, several researchers I spoke to objected to the rote conformity and intellectual passivity demanded of investigators running trials. One of the country's leading medical geneticists told me that the trial protocols are "ethically ready, we are just supposed to follow the rules." These scientists questioned the integrity of the evidence that trials produce, as "real patients are much sicker than the ideal ones of clinical trials"; and they tried to work out alternative treatment protocols for new drugs that were aggressively marketed and in high demand in the public health-care system, even though many had not yet been approved for use in the country.

As I could see in Poland and Brazil, governments, local entrepreneurs, and research centers are eager to attract pharmaceutical investments and to maintain their positions as clinical trials hubs. Host countries have proven themselves quite adaptive to business demands, and the trial enterprise, arguably, feeds upon public health institutions and resources. Industry-funded trial infrastructures also compensate for inadequately funded state research. Amid restructuring economies and unresolved conflicts over the role of the state in trade regulation and in health-care delivery, islands of clinical research and new drug markets take form. In my long-term engagement with trial entrepreneurs and researchers, I probed the adequacy of protections that are in place in the United States and elsewhere, how they are modified, and how they vary from place to place.

Some of the troubling features of the offshoring of trials are known: the ethical problems surrounding the "availability" of patients facing medical crises and poverty. Others may be less so, such as the unequal terms of trials that draw heavily from public resources but whose immediate benefits reach only a few. I also specify the kinds of harm that, despite the oversight of ethics review committees and informed consent forms, are nonetheless produced. The question of who is ultimately responsible for the experimental subject's immediate and long-term well-being is also buried beneath the "paper ethics" (Jacob and Riles 2007) of the globalized clinical trial. The absence of sustained debates over the politics of clinical research and specific pro-patient policies leaves ample room for opportunistic and self-serving behaviors. Better systems of protection, accountability, and benefit sharing are in order.[19]

Treatment Saturation

Currently, pharmaceutical sponsors are engaged in a turf war over human subjects. This competition is not only about the numbers of subjects a given company can recruit. It is also about recruiting subjects quickly. As one veteran recruiter told me at a 2003 Washington, D.C., conference on international clinical trials, "It's really a problem. I don't know anybody who has really cracked the code. Sometimes you get lucky and you fill the study quickly, but for the most part, patients are really difficult to find, and they are difficult to find because everybody is looking for them."

What drives the demand for larger pools of human subjects? First, it is the sheer number of clinical trials being run. The advent of blockbuster drugs with sales of more than a billion dollars annually (such as Prozac, Lipitor, Nexium, and Viagra) has led to the profitable and highly competitive "me-too" drugs business. With minimal pharmacological alteration, me-too drugs build on or mimic blockbuster drugs and exploit well-established markets. Trials for me-too drugs require large numbers of patients and often produce little or no evidence of additional therapeutic gain.[20]

Second, it is the need for larger subject cohorts. To satisfy U.S. regulatory demands regarding the long-term safety of a new drug, clinical trials must include greater numbers of patients, especially in the case of drugs designed to be widely prescribed. "If a few years ago you needed five hundred people to make a better aspirin, today you need five thousand," a regulatory affairs officer for Tem/po told me. "Three adverse events in a population of three thousand are enough for the Food and Drug Administration to tell you that you need more research. The bigger the population you have tested up front, the better your chances of speeding the drug's regulatory approval."

Third, it is the rapid growth of particular therapeutic classes. Some classes like lipid regulators, antidepressants, acid pump inhibitors, and oncologics are expanding as new and competitor compounds are being developed concomitantly. The race to be the first to get drugs approved and marketed steps up the search for human subjects. In the words of a medical affairs executive at AR/CH, "When a therapeutic class gets hot, it's like a cattle stampede [for trial participants]." Fourth, there is significant growth in the number of new chemical entities—patents are inundating the U.S. Patent Office for compounds that have yet to undergo clinical testing (CenterWatch 2005).

Changes in the science of drug development also impact subject recruitment. As researchers develop new and more complex molecules, more human experiments are taking place to determine their clinical and market viability. As a CRO executive put it to me, "There is nothing worse than killing a drug late." According to his scientific adviser, animal testing no longer provides adequate filtering, and the drug industry is investing heavily in early Phase 1 human trials.[21] "It used to be that 90 percent of the novel compounds got filtered out in animal testing. Now that rate is dropping to below 50 percent. This is partly due to the fact that there are more therapeutic targets. But it is also because we can't filter things out preclinically as we used to, such as toxicity, for example. More and more compounds enter human testing, yet "fewer and fewer make it into Phase 3 trials," he added.[22] "You might be able to make better laboratory mice, but the real guinea pigs will be human."

Finally, the available pool of human subjects in major Western pharmaceutical markets is shrinking.[23] We are using too many drugs. And this "treatment saturation" is making Americans and Western Europeans increasingly unusable from a drug-testing standpoint. As one of the pioneers of the clinical trials industry put it to me: "People live on pills in the West. You have the fifty-year-old who takes four or five different medications. Someone living in Eastern Europe may be on one medication for high blood pressure or whatever, but certainly not four or five." In other words, our pharmaceuticalized bodies produce too many drug-drug interactions. We are less and less capable of showing specific drug effectiveness, making test results more ambiguous and thus less valuable.[24]

Curiously, while from an industry standpoint the pool of human subjects in the United States has been shrinking, in the last two decades medical reformers have strongly pushed for the inclusion of underrepresented groups (based on sex and gender, race and ethnicity, and age) in scientific research. This came along with the mobilization of patient advocacy groups around AIDS and other life-threatening diseases, for example, to demand access to experimental therapies (Epstein 1996).[25] Medical reformers have questioned the generalizability of biomedical data, arguing that variation contributes to disease vulnerability and treatment outcomes. Federal initiatives have been launched to encourage or mandate the inclusion of representatives of designated subgroup populations in research so as to make it more relevant. In his landmark study *Inclusion*, sociologist Steven Epstein shows that the institutionalization of the U.S. inclusion-and-difference paradigm has led, among other things, to a biological reification of identity categories, thus drawing attention away from the inequalities that are rooted not in biology but in society (2007:281).

While the National Institutes of Health have mandated diversity in clinical trials, it is less clear how the industry has interpreted this policy of inclusion and how it is taken up in offshore research. In 1998, the FDA issued the Demographic Rule, which requires trial sponsors to tabulate the number of subjects enrolled in studies on the basis of gender, race, and age, as well as to analyze safety and effectiveness data by demographic subgroup. Other nonbinding guidance documents encourage sponsors to analyze modifications of dose or dosage intervals for specific subgroups.[26] One scientist, for example, described her company's Russian research population as age-diverse and asserted that this diversity facilitated drug approval: "Different pollution profiles, different ways of regulating (or not regulating) air pollution, and high rates of lung cancers and respiratory diseases mean shorter life spans. There you have people getting cancer who are a lot younger. Younger people are more desirable from the perspective of trials because they are a better bet to be responsive to a therapy. And we have more data up-front for different age groups, which is good for approval." Here, the rhetoric of diversity appears to shore up a lucrative (and seemingly open-ended) search for subjects, themselves trapped in sick environments and highly unequal power relations, but who meet criteria for regulatory approval and marketing plans. For many of my industry contacts, the rhetoric of such operational efficiency trumped the rhetoric of diversity. Through strategic protocol design and subject selection criteria, the industry deploys a trial science that, in Epstein's words, "may swamp any differences potentially detectable between subgroups" (2007:285).[27]

Regardless of how many Americans are ready to become trial subjects, the pool will never be large enough to satisfy the current level of demand in pharmaceutical research. Regulatory considerations and calculations of cost-effectiveness continue to play a crucial role and are pushing the research enterprise to other shores. In 2004, the FDA registered 542 new commercial clinical research "starts," as measured by how many commercial investigational new drug (IND) application submissions the agency received.[28] Poland, a country with a population one-eighth that of the United States, registers an average of 400 new commercial trials annually. The neighboring Czech Republic averages 300. A chemist (whom I shall call Martin), a leader in the Czech trial industry, explained to me in 2005 that since that country has one of the highest rates of colon cancer in the world, it has become "a hub for colon cancer studies." In most cases, data from such trials will be used to gain approval from the FDA or from the European Agency for the Evaluation of Medicinal Products (EMEA). He said that people who live outside major pharmaceutical markets enroll in these trials "to access state-of-the-art technology."[29] Martin estimated that one in one hundred Czech citizens (or some 100,000 people) had at some point participated in clinical trials, which are now, from his point of view, becoming less of an exceptional domain and "a normal part of health-care delivery."

✦◇✦

The four-phase approach to drug testing was implemented on the heels of the scandal over thalidomide, a drug that was found to cause severe birth defects.[30] In 1962, in response to the crisis, the U.S. Congress mandated that all new drug applications submitted to the FDA should be based on "adequate and well-controlled investigations." The industry's legal challenge to the FDA's new authority to analyze the efficacy of pre-1962 drugs "delayed implementation of these regulations" (Marks 1997:128). By 1970, the agency adopted the randomized controlled trial as the gold standard for assessing the safety and efficacy of new therapies. Participants in clinical trials were to be randomly assigned to treatment or control arms of a study. Randomization reduces differences among groups by equally assigning people with certain characteristics among all the trial arms. The procedure aims at minimizing bias of selection and affords investigators and statisticians greater confidence in clinical trials results, that is, a greater likelihood that the effects of an intervention are linked to that intervention and not to some other cause. As historian Harry Marks points out in *The Progress of Experiment*, reformers promoted this statistical "new impersonal device" as a way of controlling "physicians' enthusiasm for new treatments" and limiting business interests in medicine (ibid.:12; also see Meldrum 1994).

Yet new scientific and statistical specialists were required to carry out "adequate and well-controlled clinical investigations," as one contract research organization executive recollected. "Particularly academic scientists," he said, were ill-prepared to design and carry out trials in accordance with the new and strict regulatory rules. Just as animal toxicological testing had become a business subspecialty in drug development in the previous decade, so now would human testing. This executive became an expert in the new regulatory science where others lacked the know-how or capacity. The premium was on patient uniformity, as he put it, "to achieve uniformity of study subjects to make sure that the patient population was as uniform as possible" and thus reduce the number of variables affecting results.

Prisons became the pharmaceutical industry's trial destination of choice. After a few years, however, this golden era of wide-scale prisoner testing would be denounced and severely limited (Hornblum 1999; Moreno 2000). Indeed, the scale of prison-based research was impressive. An estimated 90 percent of drugs licensed in the United States prior to the 1970s were first tested on prison populations (Harkness 1996; ACHRE 1996). In 1980, the U.S. Department of Health and Human Services banned the use of prisoners for particular phases of drug testing, and the industry lost a major source of human volunteers. But by then, it had shifted a good deal of its research elsewhere—namely, to countries such as England and Sweden where "regulation did not necessarily hinder initiating trials." The drug industry was now routinely outsourcing laboratory and clinical research, and contract research organizations were expanding their work.

By the early1990s, drug development had become a globalized endeavor, in part under the aegis of the International Conference on Harmonisation of Technical Requirements for Registration of Pharmaceuticals for Human Use, known as the ICH, in which the Food and Drug Administration played a key initiating role. This project brought regulatory authorities from the United States, Western Europe, and Japan together with industry experts. The ICH created international standards to ensure that high-quality and safe drugs would be developed and registered in the most efficient and cost-effective way. The Good Clinical Practice (GCP) was defined in the ICH as an international ethical and scientific quality control standard for assuring the protection of subjects and credibility of data. ICH-GCP aimed to expedite safe and effective human testing and to prevent the unnecessary duplication of clinical trials. Most importantly for the clinical trials industry, ICH-GCP standards made clinical data from international research sites transferable and acceptable to regulatory bodies in these major markets.[31] It also would make it easier for a new drug to be registered by different countries and marketed globally.

As sociologist John Abraham notes, there was an intricate political economy to this drive to standardize testing requirements internationally. "Drug regulatory agencies had come under intense pressure to accelerate their regulatory review process, but typically without commensurate additional resources from their governments. . . . The industry strove to decrease the cost and duration of R&D by reducing regulatory requirements imposed by the state and to reach larger markets more effectively." Even though international harmonization emphasized patient safety, the standards adopted by ICH "relaxed the extent to which trials might detect safety problems" (2007: 48–49).

Today, contract research organizations are highly competitive transnational businesses running clinical trials for pharmaceutical, biotechnology, and medical device firms; their growth is projected to be faster than pharmaceutical industry growth (Parexel 2005:35). The CRO industry claims that it employs roughly 40 percent of the clinical research personnel involved in drug development.[32] In selecting a CRO, pharmaceutical sponsors weigh the cost of a study, its quality, and its timeliness. In the words of one executive, "We recruit patients quickly and more cheaply than academic medical centers. We know the regulations of investigational procedures in various countries, the time it takes for studies to be approved and launched, and the market possibilities there."

Most CROs are involved in locating research sites, recruiting patients, and, in some cases, drawing up the study design and performing analyses. Sometimes they work directly with primary health-care facilities, hospitals, or consortia of therapeutic specialists. Some even have their own centralized institutional review boards (IRBs). IRBs are, ideally, independent boards composed of scientific and nonscientific members who review protocols and subject enrollment methods to ensure the safety of trial volunteers.[33] Elements considered in the cost-effective siting of trials include population disease profiles, mortality rates, levels of local unemployment, per-patient trial costs, and potential for future marketing of the drug to be approved. CROs investigate the host country's regulatory environment and consider the nature of health-care coverage. They look at the efficacy of local ethical review boards, recruit experts, and gauge outlooks and regulations on the use of placebos, for example.

In the context of global trials, the statistical bias-reduction strategy of the randomized approach is applied, but it is also circumvented. There is now bias induction in the design of protocols and in the recruitment of convenient populations, as one clinical trials expert told me: "In my recruitment strategy, I can use subject inclusion criteria that are so selective that I can 'engineer out' the possibility of adverse events being seen. Or I can demonstrate that my new drug is better by 'engineering up' a side effect in another drug [by doubling its dose, for example]. . . . That is the big game of clinical trials."

In 2004, the International Committee of Medical Journal Editors (ICMJE) began a movement for trial registration, that is, to ensure that "information about the existence and design of clinically directive trials was publicly available" (Laine et al. 2007:2734). Clinical trials data are typically highly edited; negative or neutral results can be suppressed. The editors initiated a policy requiring investigators to deposit information about trial design into an accepted clinical trials registry before patient enrollment begins. But the "big game"—beyond the known problem of selective reporting of trial results—almost ensures that severe risks go undetected during clinical trials, and "it is not clear how transparency in the reporting of results can be achieved if a sponsor chooses to represent its products in the best possible light" (Psaty and Kronmal 2008:1817). Reform advocates call for more independence of investigators and a wider scrutiny of the design of protocols

(DeAngelis et al. 2004, 2005). Often employing biased samples and unable to detect uncommon but potentially fatal drug reactions, trials are producing highly manipulated and less therapeutically significant evidence, they argue. Deborah Zarin and colleagues note what is at stake: "Future volunteers are at risk for being misled and harmed when their consent and the trial design are not fully informed by prior research" (2007:912).

One senior scientist at AR/CH is keenly aware of both the scientific and legal ramifications of these critiques. As for the science of drug development, she says, "the process has no credibility left." In her company, she heads a triage committee with other physicians. They review pharmaceutical research protocols and decide which ones their company should pursue and bid on. The era when CROs were "just handed a protocol" and carried it out without "really understanding it" is over, she told me. The pool of subjects for trials is more and more "biologically edited," to use her phrasing.[34] "We are seeing many more protocols with subject inclusion and exclusion criteria that are too difficult to meet, like advanced untreated diabetes," she said. Colleagues avoided bidding on some of these trials "because it is too dangerous and costly for us to monitor patients. The experiment becomes too difficult to control on the ground."

As I learned in my study, CROs have different standards and operating procedures with respect to accepting and implementing risky protocols and different levels of toleration for potential liabilities. Researchers at AR/CH also felt that the biases built into recruitment strategies and protocol design were increasing chances that ineffective and unsafe drugs would gain FDA approval. They said that they were educating pharmaceutical clients to be more safety conscious and realistic in their expectations and demands. Indeed, the global expansion of clinical trials goes hand in hand with new evidence-making strategies that carry, alongside prospective medical benefits, their own forms of risk.

Experimentality

I started thinking about this study as I was concluding my research on the Chernobyl nuclear disaster in Ukraine. The scale of Chernobyl and its long-term effects have been subjects of bitter scientific dispute and political wrangling. In *Life Exposed* (2002), I showed how a catastrophe whose scale was unimaginable and difficult to map became manageable through a particular dynamic of "nonknowledge." By delaying public announcement of the disaster, suppressing data on casualties and immediate danger, forging limited parameters of biological risk, and legally filtering out emerging ill-ness claims, state policy makers exacerbated the public health problems they tried to resolve and generated new ones. The sort of experimentation unleashed in this medical disaster exceeded the logistical capacities of any single agency or state to bring it under control. How knowledge production about it advanced or slowed was itself the result of scientific and political negotiation that, in the end, gave citizens few stable resources to act on in their efforts to secure compensation from the state.

The global clinical trial is a large-scale and multivariable process; uncer-tainties pervade its inputs and outputs. One clinical researcher told me, for example, that in clinical trials it is not just that adverse events are insuffi-ciently reported, but that harm is "generally underhypothesized." Such un-derhypothesizing does not necessarily mean deliberate suppression of ad-verse events. Rather it reflects logistical incapacities of the trial operational model and of the system of modern drug regulation that created it. We have seen the story of missed or underreported harms before, be it related to a widely marketed cholesterol-lowering statin, an antiarthritic, an anti-depressant, or an antidiabetic drug. I am intrigued by the temporality of these harm stories—involving suppression of critical data and warning signs, media exposure of manipulations in the drug trial phase, and on-going legal battles over compensation and remediation—and with the state-market complicities that they reveal.

My work on Chernobyl and this work have attuned me to a social and scientific reality beyond the more traditional notion of the experiment as a "singular, well-defined instance embedded in the elaboration of a theory and performed in order to corroborate or to refute certain hypotheses" (Rheinberger 1995:109). Citizens who claimed to be "exposed" (be it to ion-izing radiation or to a harmful drug) were led into open-ended experimen-tal processes that were essentially beyond their consent. At stake in their enrollment is the *breakdown* in consent processes and in citizens' trust in state systems of regulatory and public health expertise. The issue of human subjects protection moves beyond scripted procedural issues of informed consent and into the question of legal capacities and the aggregate human conditions of which they are generative (Marks 2000). The open-endedness of Chernobyl, for example, affected more than 3.5 million people in Ukraine alone. Research clinics and nongovernmental organizations medi-ated an informal economy of disease and claims to what I called a *biological citizenship*—a massive demand for but selective access to a form of social welfare based on scientific and legal criteria that acknowledge injury and compensate for it. Such struggles over a biological citizenship took place in a context of fundamental losses related to employment and state protections against inflation, widespread corruption, and a corrosion of legal and political categories. Distributional issues were closely related to the "science" of Chernobyl. The very framing of injury was intimately associated with the region's economic restructuring, with often tragically and unjustly varying degrees of success and failure.

With the growing number of clinical trials, citizens are looking beyond the state to safeguard their health. Their particular characteristics make them resources visible not only to the state but to capital as well. The trial protocols that my interlocutors bid on are themselves products of state-mediated data requirements. Without such requirements there would be no market in CROs and no demand for human subjects. Biological citizenship, in which the very idea of citizenship is charged with the superadded burden of survival, also multiplies a new and somewhat time-sensitive resource—in the first instance, a citizen who has lost confidence in state forms of protection and who is looking for other, however temporary, ones. The "progress of experiment" (and the regulatory and financial considerations it is tethered to) depend on these market-mediated biological citizens and their consent. Assaults on health are the coinage through which the proliferating figure of the biological citizen stakes claims for biomedical resources. But what is engineered out of this global system as it is being currently deployed? Does it let health authorities off the hook and limit other sorts of interventions? Are progressive regimes of ethics, regulation, and law, in various locales, reengendering biological citizenship? What is happening to the human right to health? I will return to these issues throughout the book, and especially in chapter 4, where I consider access to high-cost drugs and the judicialization of health in Brazil.

In my fieldwork in state-run research clinics and hospitals and among Chernobyl sufferers, I observed a rapid growth in the dispensation and use of imported pharmaceuticals. Public attitudes toward health and treatment were changing. The healing powers attributed to Western drugs were immense. In Soviet times, citizens, mainly elites, who could travel to the West were often put on missions by desperate relatives and friends to procure certain medications. There was widespread distrust of doctors and of Soviet-made medicines, particularly in the face of chronic and life-threatening diseases.

Vitalii, for example, whom I met during an initial trip to Ukraine in 1992, was very preoccupied with the idea that he had prostate cancer. He asked me to bring back specific medications for him upon my next visit to

Kyiv, even though his medical records did not indicate the disease. The fact that I couldn't deliver on his order was grounds enough for him to end our conversation. I also recall the glossy blue boxes with packets of Prozac samples locked up in glass cabinets in the Chernobyl clinics, potent displays of new medical commodities. The power of the low-status Soviet physician grew exponentially as he became the gatekeeper of new healing technologies. These packets were also routinely sold among the patients I knew.

I also recall a particular lavatory in the neurological ward of the Radiation Research Center where I worked among physicians who tended to Chernobyl sufferers. It was stuffed with drugs (many were expired) and medical supplies donated by manufacturers and philanthropic organizations. Donors of these gifts obtained tax deductions and were spared the cost of properly disposing of drugs they could not sell in the West. Doctors and nurses told me that they scrounged for medical materials at local train and bus stations when they arrived. Yet this medical philanthropy was a mixed blessing. Dr. Artem Borovsky, my key interlocutor in the neurological ward, said that many doctors worked in a trial-and-error fashion to learn about these drugs' effectiveness and proper dosages, and that many patients used them improperly. Such was the face of the incipient Western pharmaceutical market in Ukraine: samples, humanitarianism, and drug "dumping" now coexisted with a discredited Soviet pharmacopeia, yielding one large uncontrolled experiment in cobbled-together access and unregulated consumption. Experiments piled upon experiments.

Dr. Borovsky and his colleagues told me how eager they were to secure clinical trial contracts. His team specialized in the diagnosis of functional disorders of the higher nervous system such as stroke, brain damage, schizophrenia, and posttraumatic stress, and it wanted to participate in industry-sponsored research for relevant treatments. Untreated diseases abounded there and the scientific infrastructures on which these researchers were dependent were rapidly deteriorating in the absence of new state funding. This combination of an ongoing public health crisis and the needs and interests of local scientific communities was leading to a reconceptualization of patients and their value. The scientific rush to rethink patients as a population with specific biological resources to be brokered in the pharmaceutical market was palpably there (Geertz 2001:21). These physician-researchers were looking just across the border, to Poland, where clinical trials were beginning to thrive in the public health-care system, and new careers and research possibilities were on the horizon. They were hoping and anticipating that the clinical trials wave would reach them soon.

When Experiments Travel reflects my continued interest in experiments and health, knowledge and power dynamics, the reconfiguration of populations as objects of governmentality, and the relations between the local and the global—this time under the rubric of a dramatically expanded globalized clinical research enterprise. A distinct modus operandi that I call experimentality supports the global drug market. Decentralized and diffused in character, this experimentality does not lend itself easily to prevailing tools of accountability. Regulated state withdrawals make it possible, favoring economic interests over empowered systems of regulatory oversight—even if only for a certain time period. In this local and time-sensitive niche of global capital, entrepreneurs, health professionals, and research subjects negotiate their own immediate stakes—for data, revenue, and therapeutic chances. Experiments draw from public resources and are coined as social goods. They are not only hypothesis-testing instruments; they are operative environments that redistribute public health resources and occasion new and often tense medical and social fields. The role of medical care—how to dispense it and whom it includes—is in question, and the line between what counts as experimentation and what counts as medical care is in flux.

The clinical trials industry sees Eastern Europe as a particularly good recruitment site. Postsocialist health-care systems are conducive to running efficient trials because they have remained centralized, and they have skilled researchers and functioning scientific infrastructures. In other words, "They are perfect platforms for clinical research," as the director of a Russian-based contract research organization put it to me in 2005. Given the unmet demand for specialized care, patient enrollment tends to be quick. High literacy rates in this region mean that subjects offer more "meaningful" informed consent, thus minimizing problems in a possible FDA audit.

Large Latin American cities such as Buenos Aires and São Paulo are also considered premium sites because, as another clinical researcher claimed, "Populations are massive. It's a question of how many patients I can get within a limited area, which reduces travel expenses." According to him, companies battle over "who gets those patients, whom I can sign up to be in my alliance so that when I do attract a pharmaceutical sponsor, I can say, 'I can line up five hundred cancer patients for you tomorrow morning.' You are seeing that happening a lot because recruitment is one of the most time-consuming and expensive portions of the process." When I asked this re-

searcher how he would respond to the critique that subject recruitment strategies were exploitative, he argued that trial expansion has had overall "positive effects" as experiments themselves have become social goods: "We provide health care where there is none and medical relief for participants."[35]

The increasing "choice" of citizens in transitioning economies to become
experimental subjects parallels their poverty status and often reveals the
limits of local standards of care and the failure of states to protect citizens.
We might know something about the formal aspects of a study, but we lack
systematic knowledge of how protection actually works, which circumstances make the trial enterprise mobile, and the real value that the patient
brings to the drug. "There are so many places that we can work in," one CRO
executive told me, suggesting that it is easy for the industry to "bypass it
altogether"—that is, local demands—and to venue-shop for hospitable environments that can maximize the sponsors' own benefit ratios in trial
agreements.

As the formal rules and regulations are adhered to, what happens beyond
rules and regulations can remain problematic—even for the conscientious
researcher who makes every effort to comply with research regulations:
"There is very tight control over what the written documents say, and that's
the ethics," one clinical trial manager told me. "As far as potential benefit or
potential harm, that does not translate into what's verbally communicated."
Critics of these highly mobile regimes focus heavily on procedural issues—
clinical conduct and informed consent—as if harm could be located exclusively within a traditional model of physician-induced neglect. The FDA's
oversight mechanisms reinforce this narrow purview despite changing practices and conflicting interests.[36] Through auditing (or its threat), the agency
holds investigators "clearly and directly accountable for conducting research ethically and liable for errors and negligence related to oversight responsibilities."[37] Trial sponsors structure their research operations around
such narrow purviews and their trials industry counterparts are free to
globally roam.

Practice overwhelms ethics in terms of who controls international guidelines for ethical research and their capacity to protect the rights, interests,
and well-being of human subjects globally.[38] With the focus on procedural
issues, anthropologist-physician Arthur Kleinman has pointed to a "dangerous break" between bioethics—an abstract philosophical discourse
grounding a set of codified norms for medical research—and empirical reality (1999). Social scientists have echoed his view by arguing that the ethics
committee model for monitoring the conduct of research turns the ethical

universe in which researchers operate into a document- and liability-driven one. Others argue that "bureaucracies of virtue" (Bosk 2007) can deflect attention from structural circumstances that can contribute to increased risk and injustice, insulating researchers from the broader contexts of inequality in which they work.[39]

Industry and regulatory concerns about ethics seem to matter primarily at the level of the data production—more specifically, in terms of ensuring the "integrity" of data. Why invest in a foreign site if one is uncertain whether the data gathered there will even be usable in the U.S. drug approval process? Was there informed consent? Did the local investigator agree to accept all responsibility in cases of harm? Did the local ethical review board examine and approve the protocol? At stake is the construction of an airtight documentary environment ensuring the portability of clinical data from anywhere in the world to U.S. regulatory settings of drug approval.

In my ethnographic work with various professionals within the contract research organization (CRO) community (including company founders and clinical trials managers), the physicians with whom CROs contract, and pharmaceutical consultants and regulators in various countries, I came to see that the global dynamics of drug production play an important role in shaping contexts in which ethical norms and delineations of human subjects change. As instances of misconduct and harm in research are exposed in the media, we must also confront questions of how populations are brought into experimental orders and the ways in which available discourses and protective mechanisms are unable to assist these groups and effectively intervene.

I also discovered an ethical variability at work in the globalization of trials, as one of several modes assisting pharmaceutical sponsors in mobilizing much larger populations of human subjects and in doing so much more quickly (Petryna 2005). Ethical variability refers to how international ethical guidelines (informed by principles and guidelines for research involving human subjects) are employed as the search for global research subjects expands. That international standardized ethics has starkly failed to account for local contexts and lived experience has become a truism in the anthropological critique of international health policy (Das 1999; Cohen 1999; Biehl 2007; Nichter 2008). In an industrial pharmaceutical context, ethical variability evolves as a tactic informing the regulation and organization of commercial clinical trials. It takes the realities of different local contexts and capacities as a given and as a basis on which to consolidate a cost-effective variability in human research.

Ethical guidelines on the ground are "workable," as one researcher told me. While the principle of workability is not explicit in research regulation, it is in many senses at work in the United States and elsewhere (see chapter 2).[40] To be sure, researchers in low- and middle-income countries must comply with regulatory and ethical standards, even "overcomply," as one Polish researcher put it, to maintain their country's pivotal role in the clinical trial market (see chapter 3). But there is a public policy vacuum with regard to how the ethical is delimited in different locales, and of how risks circulate in this new global enterprise. Capturing a dimension of ethics beyond its universal and regulatory (or normative) frameworks, I engage ethics as a field of action for anthropological inquiry. Gathering different materials (media, legal briefs, government reports) and points of view, I also address instances of contestation over the terms of clinical trials undertaken locally. In all, I point to the deep tensions of promoting equal standards for all research and in altering those standards to fit certain values and needs.[41]

Physician-anthropologist Paul Farmer has argued that in transnational medical research, "[s]ocial context is not merely local, nor are standards of care. In studies linking developed and less-developed countries, context is transnational, and such research is a reminder that some populations are not really developing but rather are being left behind by the same economic processes that enable powerful [institutions] to do research in poor countries" (2002:1266). Farmer urges us to think about the ethics of transnational medical research from a human rights and equity perspective. In order to do so we need to sustain public debate and scrutinize the myriad state-market mechanisms and scientific paradigms through which experimentality is made possible: What constitutes therapeutic significance and innovation in drug development? Which economic and scientific interests are favored, and what is the value of systems of protection? What is the normative power of national law and international guidelines?

Ethics as "Workable Document"

The controversy over placebo use in Africa in 1994 during trials of short-course AZT treatment to halt perinatal transmission of HIV is widely considered a watershed in the debate over ethical standards in global clinical research.[42] It is worth considering it as a watershed of a different sort: in how a cost-effective consolidation of variability in standards overtook efforts to make key ethical guidelines for human subjects research applicable worldwide. Underpinning this process is a more general dynamic of how new

subject populations are forged at the intersection of regulatory deliberation, commercial interests, and crises (upon crises) of public health. My
specific angle into the debate centers on how the ability of the drug industry to recruit global subjects was strengthened.

In this well-known case, some U.S. researchers argued that giving less
than the known standard-of-care therapy to those on the placebo arm of the
study was ethically responsible.[43] A placebo is an inactive treatment made
to resemble real treatment; it amounts to no treatment. Critics viewed
the use of a placebo arm in this context as highly unethical. Research in developing countries, they contended, was being held to a different standard
than that in the developed world. Marcia Angell (2000), for example, said
that practices like the use of a placebo arm were reminiscent of the Tuskegee
experiment, in which for decades the U.S. Public Health Service withheld
standard treatments from a large group of African American men infected
with syphilis so that scientists could observe the "natural" course of these
patients' untreated disease.[44]

Leaders of the U.S. National Institutes of Health and the U.S. Centers for
Disease Control, which among other government institutions authorized
and funded the AZT trial, claimed that the experiment was ethically sound
(Varmus and Satcher 1996). They cited local cultural variables and deteriorated health services as making the delivery of the best standard of care in-
feasible. It would be a paternalistic imposition, they argued, for critics in the
United States to determine the appropriate design of medical research in a
region undergoing such stress. Moreover, it was within the jurisdiction of
local and national authorities to decide the appropriate research conduct
and treatment distribution.[45]

Ethical imperialism or ethical relativism? These were the terms of the debate. The first position builds its case on histories of marginalized communities that were coerced or misled into experiments and greatly suffered as
a result. Historians point to other communities, such as those of "cooperative" patients and professional guinea pigs, that complicate these histories
of coercion (Marks 2002; Abadie 2009). The second position relativizes ethical decision making as a matter of sound "locally sensitive" science, but it
fails to consider the uptake of this relativizing move by the research enterprise itself. For me, the fact of the AZT trial—and the debates that followed
it—highlights the role of crisis in the consideration of differences in ethical
standards in the area of human research: crisis conditions frequently legitimate variability in ethical standards.[46] Historically, some crises have led,
perhaps inescapably, to experimentation.[47] But today one can, and must,

ask: Are crises states of exception or are they the norm? To what extent does the language of crisis become instrumental, granting legitimacy to experimentation when it otherwise might have none?

The debate over the ethics of the AZT trial prompted the sixth revision of the Helsinki declaration, first issued in 1964. The declaration provides guidelines for biomedical research in humans. The 2000 revision reiterates a position against placebo use when standards of treatment are known: "The benefits, risks, burdens, and effectiveness of a new method should be tested against those of the best current prophylactic, diagnostic, and therapeutic methods. This does not exclude the use of placebo, or no treatment, in studies where no proven prophylactic, diagnostic, or therapeutic method exists."[48] The ethics of the declaration was unambiguous, but its regulatory weight was not. Pharmaceutical companies, already eagerly expanding operations abroad and calculating the economic advantages of placebo use, began scrambling to learn from regulators about the legal enforceability of the declaration and finding ways to continue using the placebo. They had a strong incentive: placebos lower costs, and, many argue, placebo trials produce better evidence.[49]

Dr. Robert Temple, then director of the Center for Drug Evaluation at the FDA, undercut the regulatory significance of the Helsinki declaration and threw his support behind placebo advocates.[50] He cited the International Conference on Harmonisation's Good Clinical Practice (ICH-GCP) guideline. This guideline states, "Whether a particular placebo controlled trial of a new agent will be acceptable to subjects and investigators when there is a known effective therapy is a matter of patient, investigator, and IRB judgment, and acceptability may differ among ICH regions. *Acceptability could depend on the specific trial design and population chosen*" (2002:213—my emphasis). In other words, in spite of public outrage and a revised declaration, the ethical standard for human research amounted to variability in standards of care, a variability legitimated by the guidelines articulated by first-world regulatory agencies and industry associations.

Temple supported the placebo trial, he explained, out of concern over the quality of scientific data. But his reaction was also indicative of how state-market actors can influence the definition of experimental groups. The alternative to the placebo-control trial is the active-control trial. In an active-control trial (in which a new drug is compared with a standard one), there is an increased chance of "study defects" that arise from external factors and that might invalidate the data—such as poor patient compliance, diagnostic inconsistencies, and patients' use of concomitant medications that can obscure effect of the experimental drug. These factors, Temple asserted, can be "fatal to a trial designed to show a difference" (2002:222; see also Pocock 2002:244–245). Following this logic, subjects with no prior treatment for a particular ailment are the preferred subjects. That they are often poor and supposedly do not have access to diagnoses and treatments is precisely what makes these individuals the most "foolproof" and valuable research subjects.

Members of the clinical trials industry were keenly interested in the outcome of the debate.[51] A market strategist who worked for a contract research organization in Eastern Europe told me in 2001 that the FDA's response to the Helsinki declaration revision "made research efficiency a priority, and this was in line with what the industry wanted." Researchers could bypass the murky ethics of placebo use by providing what is known as "equivalent medication"—not necessarily the best or standard treatment, but whatever is available as a best local equivalent. "Do I give them a sugar pill or vitamin C?" this professional ironically asked. In short, the study will be ethical, the data will have integrity, and unfortunately (in this case) the patient will remain untreated. This strategist suggested that in industry-sponsored research, ethics is a workable document: "Equivalent medication in Eastern Europe is not the same as equivalent medication in Western Europe, so you could work the Helsinki declaration."

In tracing the relation between regulation and the evolution of ethical standards in human research, Harry Marks notes, "It is as if ethical discourse and the regulations governing research exist in two parallel universes which share some common elements but do not connect" (2000:14). I would argue that the aftermath of the 1994 AZT trials demonstrates how connected those universes actually are, and how transnational regulatory debates are implicated in the emergence of "local" and differentiated experimental terrains. In zones of crisis, protection and safety considerations are at times weighed against immediate health benefits or the scientific knowledge to be gained. Ethics and method are thus modified to fit the local context and experimental data required.

In a 2004 study, David Kent and colleagues reviewed 73 randomized clinical trials carried out during or after 1998 in sub-Saharan Africa in three clinical domains of high public health relevance: HIV disease, tuberculosis treatment, and malaria prophylaxis. The findings show how minimal an impact the debate over the ethics of the AZT trials and the Helsinki declaration revision have had on applications of research guidelines and standards of care. Of the 65 trials that reported funding sources, 42 received at least some funding from a Western governmental agency; 17 received funding from an international body; 14 received funding from local governments; 12 received funding from the pharmaceutical industry; and 11 received funding from private foundations (Kent et al. 2004:240). "Among studies selected in this review, only 16% of the trials conducted in resource-poor settings provided therapy that could be considered consistent with the best current standards of care, even when the Declaration of Helsinki required that standard" (ibid.:240, 241).

Consistency with best standards of care (during and after a trial) often hinges on national legislation and the steps legislators take to discourage inconsistency.[52] Some countries faced with a recent sudden growth of industry-sponsored research may have minimal bureaucracies to address adverse or catastrophic events. Neither might these governments have the political leverage or an interest in pressing for fairer procedures and access to drugs during and after trials. Thus a distinction is to be made between ethical codes (in which the definition of what constitutes biomedical harm is fairly unambiguous) and ethical regulation (in which deliberation of those definitions is balanced against economic, scientific, and regulatory constraints and demands). Ethical regulation as inscribed in public policy and law entails minimally enforceable procedures governing human research. It is also a realm of contingent practice, and the allocation of protection for human subjects is far from settled here.

In the early 1990s, a few years before the controversial AZT trials, the FDA began to actively promote the globalization of clinical trials, declaring that the search for sites and sources of data is part of its mandate to determine the safety and efficacy of new drugs. The FDA took an active role in establishing the International Conference on Harmonisation and Good Clinical Practice (ICH-GCP). Many countries that had already tailored their patent laws according to the provisions of the TRIPS (trade-related aspects of intellectual property rights) Agreement also signed on to the ICH-GCP.[53] They were eager to attract new investments and participate in the booming production of global pharmaceuticals. As ICH-GCP members, they began the costly work of setting up national agencies that could standardize and monitor the conduct and performance of trials in their territories. Countries were required to create ethical review boards to ensure the rights and protections of patients.

While the implementation of ICH-GCP guidelines varied from country to country, the number of subjects involved in international clinical trials grew enormously, from 4,000 in 1995 to 400,000 in 1999, according to partial estimates.[54] By 2001, when I began this research, the largest documented increase in clinical trials participation had occurred in Eastern Europe and Latin America (India and China are now key areas of outsourced clinical research).[55] This global growth brought with it a new set of unknowns related to the circumstances of research and concerns about possible exploitation of foreign subjects. New local institutions provided the legal and technical bare minimum for clinical trials to globalize, but large-scale regulatory frameworks for registering global clinical trials or monitoring their conduct remained limited at best. Many proposals have been made for improving the system. For instance, in 1999, the Office of Inspector General (OIG), a periodic auditor of the FDA, found that "in spite of its active promotion of the search for sites and subjects elsewhere," the FDA has not been able to protect these subjects. [56] To address this gap, the inspector general recommended that the FDA support and, in some cases, directly help to create appropriate ethical review boards.[57]

This approach involves more monitoring and more reliance on local committees, and it leans heavily toward what political scientist Iris Young called a "liability model" of accountability (2004). Let regulators name the responsible local parties (in some cases, this would mean first creating such oversight bodies) and surely those parties can gather information and make the right decisions; surely they can prevent inappropriate research. This approach presupposes a working and fair legal system (among other things). Much is also assumed about who is and is not the agent of abuse (most typically defined as the individual investigator). The fact is that certain conditions have to be met before a liability model can effectively protect research subjects. States themselves need to act as protectors and not abusers; transnational corporations need to respect the rights and dignity of all research subjects and recognize that different situations elicit different levels of coercion; and international ethics codes must be enforceable. In short, what I am pointing to is a political and ethical milieu lying beyond a procedural one governing investigator conduct.

As the rapid growth of clinical trials was under way, scandals exposed the structural flaws and absences of institutionalized protective structures in a now-globalized system. Consider Trovan, which, for a short time, was one of this country's best-selling antibiotics. But in 1999, the FDA restricted its use, as it was associated with liver damage and deaths. Before Trovan was approved for marketing in December 1997, the manufacturer wanted to widen the drug's scope of therapeutic uses. In 1996, a company researcher and his team traveled to the city of Kano, Nigeria, to test Trovan on pediatric victims of a bacterial meningitis outbreak. Nigeria was undergoing a period of massive civil unrest under the Abacha military dictatorship. Doctors Without Borders was already injecting children with a fast-acting antibiotic (ceftriaxone), proven effective for treating bacterial meningitis, at a local city hospital.

The objective of the new protocol was to show that an oral version of Trovan would work as well as or better than ceftriaxone. This protocol was not approved by a U.S. ethics committee and received inadequate review in the host country. Legal documents show that patient consent forms used in the manufacturer's defense were backdated.[58] The company team arrived at Kano Infectious Diseases Hospital and selected two hundred children who were waiting in line to receive ceftriaxone. Some of these children were given Trovan in an oral form never tested on humans before; others were given a dose of ceftriaxone at a dose lower than that of the standard of care for meningitis. The team is alleged not to have explained the experimental nature of Trovan to subjects; parents believed their children were receiving a proven treatment.[59] According to the complaint filed by a New York law firm on behalf of the parents, the lower dosage allowed company researchers to show that Trovan was more efficacious. This low dosing also, the parents claim, resulted in the deaths of eleven children.[60]

This two-billion-dollar lawsuit was one of the first cases brought by foreigners against a U.S.-based pharmaceutical company.[61] The plaintiffs' lawyers suggested that a chain of complicity made the children available for research. This chain included Nigeria's military rulers and state officials, Ministry of Health officials, and local hospital administrators; U.S. FDA regulators who authorized an unapproved drug's export to Nigeria for "humanitarian" purposes; and company researchers who, from a group of children waiting for standard treatments, selected subjects for their own trial. All were involved, lawyers claimed, in violating principles of the Nuremberg Code and other codes of human subjects protection.[62] Legal documents referred to these codes as "customary laws" that are "made up of fundamental principles of a civil society that are so widely held that they constitute binding norms on the community of nations" (*Rabi Abdullahi, et al., v. Pfizer Inc.*, 01 Civ. 8118, Plaintiffs' memorandum of law: 6).

The defendant's lawyers, by contrast, downplayed the authority of these codes and stated that they are guidelines and "are not treaties." In some U.S. cases, federal judges have indeed ruled that internationally accepted codes of human subjects protection (the Nuremberg Code and the Helsinki declaration, for example) cannot be relied on as the basis for civil suits. Company attorneys situated the research in the context of a "massive epidemic killing more than 11,000 people," and linked the epidemic outbreak to "woefully inadequate" sanitary conditions. By suggesting that their experimental treatment could only do good in such a desperate context, defense attorneys troubled the criteria marking the difference between the experimental and the therapeutic. The company contended that its researchers did no harm and, in fact, saved lives. Lawyers stated that it would be "paternalistic" for an American court to adjudicate the appropriate conduct of medical research in a country undergoing a public health crisis, thus echoing the ethically relativizing stance already familiar in the African AZT case (*Rabi Abdullahi, et al., v. Pfizer Inc.*, 01 Civ. 8118, Memorandum of law: 1).

From the brief sketch of this legal parrying, two points are worth emphasizing. First, as much as one would like to see the Kano case as an instance of the "dubious" or of the "exceptional," an interlocking set of regulatory, commercial, and state interests were at play here—a constellation of interests that can introduce uncertainty with respect to the observability of international ethics codes in local contexts or even suspend the relevance of such codes altogether.[63] In this specific case, a functional ethical review of U.S. industry-sponsored research would have been necessary and might even have prevented the tragedy. But at the site of experimentation, interests were not on the side of protection but were overwhelmingly on the side of recruitment and making vulnerable populations available to research.

Second, contextual factors (crisis and its humanitarianisms) provided a ready-made scenario for short-term biomedical research. The local public health crisis occasioned an *expedient experimentality*, giving researchers access to highly endangered and valuable subjects. [64] A discourse of lifesaving urgency masked highly questionable arrangements. But when ethics becomes a "workable document," standard consent processes erode, as does a citizen's trust in state protection. Experiments—particularly those enacted in public health crises—can be unreachable by international ethics codes.[65] The case of Trovan is still being adjudicated, but deliberations so far suggest that knowledge of wrongdoing is always contestable as legal fair play, and, even if evident, knowledge of wrongdoing does not necessarily translate into the ability to prosecute wrongdoers. The manufacturer argued that the case should be adjudicated in Nigerian courts. The Southern District of New York court has agreed, and the case continues to unfold in Nigerian courts.

Floater Sites and Hidden Harms

The growing demand for human subjects abroad cannot be understood without a knowledge of what is happening domestically in the United States. Recall that in the early 1980s, the use of prisoners for research in the United States became extremely limited, and the industry had to look for alternatives. But the continuation of prison research had strong advocates. Dr. Louis Lasagna, cofounder of the Tufts Center for the Study of Drug Development, made the case that with the eclipse of the U.S. prison-testing infrastructure, researchers were losing the ability to test for adverse reactions to drugs. Prisoners, especially recidivists, made long-term safety studies possible. Referring to the closing of a Kentucky prison-related addiction research center, Dr. Lasagna wrote, "Without such a facility, this work is unlikely to be done elsewhere, and the sick public will become the unwilling (and unconsenting) research subject of the future" (1977:2351).

What was then called liability testing (now safety testing) had been limited, and today it remains one of the least developed aspects of drug testing. Moreover, the public lacks mechanisms for evaluating the safety of drugs even after they have been put on the market. This became alarmingly clear in the recent cases of the COX-2 drugs such as rofecoxib (better known as Vioxx, shown to increase risk of heart disease) and newer antidepressant drugs (such as Paxil, now linked to a higher frequency of suicidal behavior in young adults and children).[66]

Revelations of postmarketing adverse drug effects and large numbers of lawsuits have forced companies to invest in new legal strategies to contain the cost of litigation and restore market confidence.[67] But remediation is not just a legal but also a technical matter. One of my industry contacts went further and suggested that current drug development operates on "the paradigm of expected failure." As he put it, "In any industrial system, if you spend ten times as much on repair as on prevention, you are just going to live in a continued cycle of loss. For every dollar spent on an investigation, ten dollars are spent on going back and fixing the data after the fact." An American lawyer working for a small pharmaceutical firm concurred that legal strategies tend to account for safety failures only after the fact. "Unfortunately, it takes an injury in clinical trials to figure out who is going to be responsible."[68]

Back to history. In the early 1990s, the bulk of clinical trials still occurred in academic medical settings in the United States and in Western Europe. With the "drug pipeline explosion" producing an overdemand for investigational sites and subjects, U.S. pharmaceutical companies and CROs began to tap and even to prefer private community-based medical practices and primary-care centers.[69] Physicians were eager to turn their practices into research sites. Initial interest came, in part, as a response to lowered Medicare reimbursements and changes in the structure of HMO payments. Physicians saw clinical trials as an additional source of revenue. But big profits often did not materialize, owing to the many uncompensated or hidden costs related to study start-up, the expenses of regulatory compliance, and adverse events management and reporting (Parexel 2005:125). These economics have occasioned the pervasive phenomenon of what are known as floater sites. The operators of fly-by-night investigative sites promise many patients, routinely underbid for contracts, and are not particularly concerned with achieving standards of full regulatory compliance.

Consider this story. A researcher told me that a manufacturer once approached his company to test its drug (now withdrawn from the market) for additional uses. The protocol was designed to show that the drug could treat, among other things, infections due to ruptured appendixes. The researcher explained why his CRO lost and another CRO won the contract. "Whereas we went to the tried-and-true academic sites for patient enrollment, they went to the southwestern United States, to a ring of facilities, in order to enroll trial subjects. By going to a southwestern hospital chain treating Hispanics with little or no medical insurance, this CRO far outstripped us in enrollment."

Floater sites make their money and then disappear from the clinical trials food chain. Their existence lowers the profitability of clinical research in the United States.[70] Moreover, auditing mechanisms have not expanded to meet the proliferation of floater sites; there are concerns about trial safety and the reliability of the data produced there. One very real factor pushing research to other countries is this phenomenon—whether it is to pursue more floater sites elsewhere or as an escape from the economic constraints the phenomenon imposes here. Countries like Poland, for example, bid their research services as a more reliable alternative to American floater sites.

The reality of the rescue trial adds another layer of complexity to the ways in which domestic issues affect the global movement of industry-sponsored research. The term "rescue" applies to a study that begins in one location but, because of poor recruitment, is shifted to another location midway through the trial. Some trials that were initially launched in Western Europe, for example, were shifted to Eastern European countries (which were considered "rescue countries" in the early to mid-1990s). The term can also apply to a study that takes place when the life cycle of a new drug is suddenly cut short, which requires rapid patient enrollments and a new trial launch. Rescue studies of this sort can result from unforeseen product failures (owing to adverse drug effects, for example). As I learned, both modes of rescue are a significant part of CROs' work.[71]

Hidden harms. Consider the recent troubles with Merck's blockbuster drug Vioxx. A recent meta-analysis of all Vioxx clinical trials (published in the *Lancet* in December 2004) revealed that evidence of cardiovascular risk from COX-2 inhibitors was known before September 2004, when the manufacturer withdrew the drug from the market (Juni et al. 2004). By the mid-1990s, Merck, like other companies, was beginning to offshore part of its clinical research. Vioxx underwent testing in countries such as Poland—a country that, as I mentioned earlier, has had one of the highest rates of cardiovascular-disease-related deaths in the world. In fact, in their *Lancet* analysis, Juni and colleagues suggest that contexts with different background risks can indeed lead to a misclassification or underappreciation of coronary events, which, in turn, "could have biased results in trials that did not include external appraisal of safety outcomes" (the use of study monitors, for example).[72]

In 2005, I spoke with several investigators who ran Vioxx studies overseas. Understandably perhaps, they denied any problem at their investigative sites and refused to engage in the Vioxx debate. But I sensed that this latest scandal over drug safety had made them hypersensitive about the design of studies in general. Dr. Jan Mazur (a pseudonym), who monitors AR/CH's trial sites in Eastern Europe, emphasized that studies themselves carry "background risk" owing to inadequate modeling of adverse events. In his experience, drug companies tend to choose the most cost-effective instruments to observe and record patients' symptoms, pain scales, for example, versus more costly laboratory exams. But this is not a matter of simply saving on research costs. His U.S. supervisor went further and told me that protocols generally "focus on proving efficacy" and fail to model potential harms.

This science of underhypothesizing harm can potentially strengthen as new study sites with high background risks can obscure important information about a drug's safety profile. Seen in this light, offshoring is yet another factor that can make the drug-related significance of these problems disappear. And if adverse events ever do appear in postmarketing, they can be attributed to environmental or individual causes rather than to the drug.[73] Harm, postexperiment, is difficult to prove. And the consent forms patients signed are of limited value in the face of it. These forms might document the experiment's explicit goals. What subjects generally lack is a broader and informed understanding of the scientific and economic motivations and risks driving the evidence-gathering exercise. People also lack resources to address voids in national regulation and international policy, voids that enable the uncharted expansion of experimentality that they, for their own particular reasons, choose to be a part of.

The effects of private-sector research on the welfare of large numbers of people is increasing in significance (Kahn, Mastroianni, and Sugarman 1998), but the institutional and personal benefits deriving from this expansion are unevenly distributed; they favor industry's immediate goals and do little to address research-related therapeutic misconceptions or to remediate local health inequities. Moreover, current institutional ideas about patient protection remain narrowly conceived, and ideas about harm (how it is produced in the broader contexts of experimentation) need specification amid the systematic uncertainties built into research. Ethnographic knowledge, I believe, can help subjects and local researchers to clarify expectations so that they can critically weigh participation in the research enterprise and fruitfully advocate for safer and fairer procedures.

The Aftermath of Clinical Trials

Once at the periphery of global trade, national health systems constitute emerging pharmaceutical markets. They have also arguably become cogs in the outsourced research enterprise. On the ground, clinical research and public health concerns remain largely disconnected. Academic medicine can play a vital role in bridging the gap with health technology assessment initiatives, thus becoming a resource for health policy (see chapter 4). Since 2002, I have engaged a team of academic researchers of a major university-based hospital in Brazil. The team is critical of the ways drug firms are influencing medical research and health delivery in Brazil. Industry-sponsored trials are also exercises in generating medical consensus and patient demand, thus launching new pharmaceuticals in the country without public scrutiny of their added value. They are also concerned with the uneven terms of trial agreements and patient welfare once trials are over and experimental drugs are no longer accessible.

In mending the gap between drug value and drug price, these researchers analyze the efficacy and dosage requirements of high-cost medicines that are part of the country's pharmaceutical assistance program and design alternative treatment protocols (with either altered dosages or comparable drugs). They are particularly concerned with drugs that do not provide measurable benefits aside from lowering nonclinical indicators, such as the reduced virological response promised by the hepatitis C drug peginterferon. Some of the newest drugs cost twenty times more than existing treatments and as Dr. Paulo Picon, an advocate for reform, argues, their efficacy is not much better. "The industry is pressuring the state to purchase these drugs." He went on to compare a gram of peginterferon to a gram of gold: "One gram of gold costs twenty-four dollars. Today, one gram of peginterferon costs about two million dollars . . . one gram. With this one gram you can treat 110 patients and you might prevent, you might prevent one liver cirrhosis. One cirrhosis in 110 patients . . . you *might* prevent."[74]

Brazil's progressive constitution (1988), born in the transition from military dictatorship to democratic rule, guarantees citizens the right to universal health care. Desperate patients and their families use this right to pressure regional governments to buy new drugs and drugs in the experimental stages. Many patient groups, some industry supported, have formed over the years. People lobby for their disease to become the target of a special federal program, and a growing number of patients are filing legal suits to guarantee pharmaceutical assistance. These new patient groups are modeling their efforts after the successful mobilization for universal and free access to AIDS therapies. According to anthropologist João Biehl, this combination of patient activism, pharmaceutical industry interests, and state reform is leading to "an incremental change in the concept of public health from prevention and clinical care to community based care and drugging— that is, public health is increasingly decentralized and pharmaceuticalized" (2006:223). This "pharmaceuticalization" raises vital questions about public health priorities and their financing, and the role of equity in the human right to health.

New configurations of market-driven medicine, law, and human rights lead to a hyperindividualized race for treatment access in local worlds. In their effort to ascertain the most efficacious doses for their patients, the Brazilian team engages in a kind of "reverse engineering" of privatization, applying a moral acid test to the practices that can compromise the scientific evidence base and that allow private interests to maintain their grip on public institutions.[75] They challenge the usual dichotomies between private exclusivity (of patient data, for example) and public openness. In hopes for sustained access to treatments and high-quality care, patients consent to this public health experiment. In closing the gaps between clinical research and effective health care, these researchers are also partnering with government officials and prosecutors to make sure that their alternative evidence will have legal weight and will inform health policy.

Experimentality is a complicated animal that transcends any artificial separation between the controlled conditions of testing (the "lab") and the public (the "field"). Its quality is dependent not merely on standardized compliances or techniques of data processing but on how commercial, scientific, regulatory, and ethical priorities are established (Abraham 2007:41). It creates its own measures of success that, at times, have fallen short of broader public health goals. In what follows, I probe how this multisided and locomotive phenomenon came to be and the many values that it assumes for private and public actors and local communities of need. The world is fast becoming a labyrinth of laboratories and data-producing sites, held together by dominant scientific paradigms and investments that overdetermine drug value today. This book interrogates that value and probes the creative role of the public in therapeutic innovation today.

CHAPTER TWO

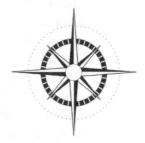

ARTS OF DRUG DEVELOPMENT

They are the mills which grinde you, yet you are
The winde which drives them.
—*John Donne*[1]

Study Mills

Across-the-Globe-Research (AGR) is located in one of several ethnically and economically diverse sections of a midwestern county. "Diversity is important for us," Evan said in a conversation in his office in 2005. The middle-aged business manager told me that there are about forty thousand clinical research sites in the country, "but only about twenty thousand are heavily involved. These sites can capture only a small percentage of the overall American population." Evan's task, in part, was to find volunteers more representative of the broader population, providing data on demographic subgroups that can enhance the drug approval process. [2] AGR is well situated to attract the range of patient types needed for its behavioral, neurological, and psychiatric trials. The area has several outpatient mental-health units affiliated with local hospital systems and a large elderly and college population in the vicinity.

The firm invests heavily in advertising. When one of my family members visited a general practitioner recently, she found leaflets from AGR placed over a stack of magazines in the waiting room. One read, "Sleep problems can be common for those with Alzheimer's disease." It had an image of a physician holding the arm of an elderly woman who is peering back at him with an expression that conveys a sense of trust. Similar leaflets sit in small piles next to automated teller machines around town, local radio programs broadcast the company's ads, and the first page of a community newspaper, available in supermarkets, cafés, and the library, consistently features an AGR ad. The advertisements for antidepressant studies feature females resembling stay-at-home mothers; those for an anxiety and sleep disorder study picture young males in dorm room–like settings. In the latter case, compensation is indicated, along with a guarantee that no reports are made to employers, schools, or insurers.

AGR is particularly keen to attract Alzheimer's patients living in the growing number of privately owned or state-subsidized senior living communities in the surroundings. The company advertises to caregivers, as they can be counted on to shuttle patients to and from study-related appointments. It promises to pay patients up to two thousand dollars for their participation. Experiments and incentives to experiment merge seamlessly into everyday life, inviting questions about how this trial nexus supplants traditional ethics of care and access and modifies health-seeking behaviors.[3]

I asked Evan to rank clinical trials from most expensive to least expensive. He was reluctant to name actual figures. Generally speaking, trial costs are based on a "cost per patient at investigator site" basis; they are usually linked to the kind of disease under study (acute infections, fatal diseases, or rare diseases versus chronic diseases), the number of medical procedures required, and the patient's insurance status.[4] Evan acknowledged that Alzheimer's trials are "at the upper end," explaining that "there are fewer patients. They are usually very sick, so there is a lot of monitoring and medical history, and you have to look at all these things. The evaluation process is very detailed and also requires high skill. As a tester I have to interpret your response and figure out if you are getting better or worse; so there's lots of expertise." Generally speaking, in the United States, "costs run between eight thousand and twelve thousand dollars per Alzheimer's patient. In Russia it is probably 40 to 50 percent cheaper."

One local doctor calls AGR a "study mill," giving a more cynical spin to Evan's statement that his company "can't take in patients fast enough." This physician witnessed the "commercial takeover" of psychiatric research within his own nearby academic medical institution and the alarming alacrity with which his colleagues took up commercially sponsored research. Yet patients, their physicians, and caregivers drive this study mill, making themselves available for this stage of drug development. Evan says his clients are not uninformed guinea pigs but have a kind of collective free will. AGR is a "freestanding research center with active populations," he says.

Slippery strategies of patient data mining, however, belie such rhetoric. "Let's say I go to the office of Dr. X," Evan told me earlier in the conversation. "He's got a huge general medicine clinic with three other doctors. That's a place you would go to for patients. They have over five thousand regular patients. The doctors can go into their files and check which patients fit the criteria of a study. They can tell a patient that 'we have this study and it looks like it would be fitting for you.'" Patient confidentiality rules would usually bar outside parties from viewing records without patient consent. But here differences between insiders and outsiders collapse. It also remains unclear to me whether these doctors are given incentives to actively enroll or refer patients, and what the nature of those incentives would be. In Russia, Evan told me, "we just ran a trial for less than half of what it was bid on in the U.S., and we did the study twice as fast. We saved our pharmaceutical client three and a half million dollars. In Russia, a doctor makes two hundred dollars a month, and he is going to make five thousand dollars per Alzheimer's patient." In this case, deteriorating health infrastructures are assigned new value as physicians-investigators position themselves in a globalizing medical market.

Dr. Sarah Coons (a pseudonym), the vice president of clinical trials operations of AR/CH, a contract research organization for which Evan had worked, told me that American doctors hesitate to refer patients to clinical trials. "Say you are an internal medicine practitioner and have a patient with a long-term chronic disease like asthma, and you refer him to a pulmonary specialist doing asthma studies. If you refer a patient for a clinical trial, you're likely to never get that patient back when the study is over. It is a loss of revenue." In her rational choice rendering, she never considers the possibility that this internist might not want to risk subjecting the patient to a nontreatment arm of a study. At any rate, Evan seemed ahead of the game, promoting clinical trial enrollment across private practices and hospitals and encouraging physicians to refer patients. He said that he was up against regulatory and infrastructural constraints: "The U.S. clinical trials system is not set up for high performance, whereas other systems are." When needed, AGR floats trial protocols to Russia. Dr. Coons's company has moved some of its operations to India, where, she says, "in ten metropolitan districts, you have the equivalent of the population of the United States."

Regulatory demands for specific types of evidence make some experiments in the United States "impossible to run," and it is Evan's task to make them possible, if not in this country, then somewhere else. He explained that one recurrent problem is the placebo-controlled trial: "The FDA likes to look at placebo-controlled studies, especially for new indications. And in the United States, if there is a comparable product [one that treats the same problem as the experimental drug] out there, it is hard to get an ethical review board to approve a placebo-control. Ethically speaking, if there is a comparable product available, then you do a comparative study. Sometimes the FDA is a bit disconnected from what the institutional review boards are willing to accept."

Evan elaborated on the fate of one impossible-to-run study that involved administering regular injections of a cancer-imaging agent to children. The product was approved for adult use, and the manufacturer wanted to have the product approved for use in children. The FDA required the manufacturer to run a trial on healthy children (aged six months to two years) to determine appropriate dosaging. "But what parent in the U.S. would put their own healthy child in a cancer-imaging agent trial?" he asked, rhetorically. American researchers rejected the study, as they believed it involved an agent "that could be detrimental to children's health." Evan then sent the protocol to his Russian colleagues. They also rejected it. "If the protocol is rejected in Russia, where does it go next?" I asked him. He said he did not know. He suspected that the agent would continue to be used "off-label"—that is, prescribed for children's use without ever being systematically studied in children.

The FDA encourages drug companies to study medical compounds in children. Under the 1997 FDA Modernization Act, a pediatric studies incentive affords certain drug applications an additional six months of patent exclusivity if a sponsor tests for a drug's safety and efficacy on pediatric populations. In some ways, the FDA's effort to generate such data is commendable. But whose children will be tested? The agency has yet to systematically investigate how its incentives and evidentiary rules are actually applied in global settings. Evan suggested that risks are measured differently depending on the location of the trial and, as his example shows, U.S. regulatory norms anticipate an unequal geography of medical access for their fulfillment. Given the challenges that U.S. drug regulation poses, location becomes a key economic decision and business asset. But is one form of inequality (lack of medical access or availability) constructing another, ethical variability? As Evan floats rejected protocols overseas, he operates in uncharted territory that also constitutes his unofficially sanctioned business niche.

I was in southern Brazil in summer 2003, when I read a local newspaper article about pediatricians in a public hospital using sildenafil (better known by its trade name Viagra) to treat children and infants with pulmonary arterial hypertension (PAH). PAH is a disease of the small pulmonary arteries. It results in a progressive increase in pulmonary vascular resistance and, ultimately, right ventricular failure and death (Humbert, Sitbon, and Simonneau 2004). Treatments including a host of medicines, oxygen, and lung transplantation alleviate symptoms of this devastating disease but do not cure it. One standard of care drug is iloprost, which in the United States can cost up to seventy thousand dollars per year and, so, is prohibitively expensive. In the absence of iloprost, local doctors were prescribing small doses of sildenafil, a drug that makes pulmonary arteries open; there was growing evidence of sildenafil's value as an addition to iloprost. The FDA had not yet reviewed the popular drug for this new indication, and doctors, there and elsewhere, were using it in an off-label way in attempts to alleviate the symptoms of PAH patients. A young pediatrician whom I met at the hospital told me that sildenafil was being used "as a last resort." Parents wanted to help their desperately sick children, and "they know we are acting in their best interest."

This situation of off-label use had other purposes too. Dr. Karin Silva (a pseudonym) explained that her "pilot study" was providing her with materials for a master's thesis. This local and informal therapeutic arrangement was also enmeshed in more formal regimes. She and colleagues were aware that the manufacturer intended to carry out multicenter trials on the secondary uses of sildenafil. They were hoping that the company would enroll their site. If the drug were shown to treat pulmonary hypertension in children (and adults), the company could extend the drug's patent. During my visit to the hospital, I also spoke with a pneumologist whom I will call Dr. Carla Bock, trained in Germany, who was attempting to formalize these trial arrangements. "We successfully treated several infants, and Pfizer has already approved us to be part of the multinational study." Yet, to Dr. Bock's dismay, her director refused to give his required permission, allegedly "out of envy and competition."

Drs. Silva and Bock are at the very desperate end of a long medical chain. They want to be involved in industry-sponsored clinical research, and they hold out hope for families with limited resources and few options. They are proud of their work; they say they want to advance science and improve care options. The off-label experiment that these doctors were tapping into sparked my curiosity about the myriad ways, formal and informal, in which drug-related data are gathered. In an effort to get a more systematic view of this process, I turned to one of the scientists responsible for the Viagra global research program. Despite the assistance of one of her senior colleagues to contact her, she did not return my phone calls or emails. When I called her colleague again, he told me that the scientist and her team would be unavailable until the company's restructuring of its international clinical research operations was completed.

This case highlights how local experimental sites evolve and are, in an indirect or haphazard way, enrolled in the globalized trial. Local research contexts influence evaluations of risks versus benefits of a given study. The availability or lack of the best standard of care can overdetermine what is accepted as the medically or morally sound thing to do. Dr. Silva and Dr. Bock point to research collaboration whose existence depends less on formal rules than on intractable inequities of access and serendipitous local decision making. National oversight bodies may not be able to keep track of this inchoate world of local protoexperiments. This case also suggests that in drug development and marketing, trial sponsors have tacit recourse to these local sites in achieving evidentiary and commercial aims.

Off-label experiments connect local medical worlds—their scientific aspirations and medical needs—with larger corporate actors and interests. They are also spin-offs of evolving drug regulation and patent regimes. This medical and commercial field of activity cuts across different and vastly unequal contexts. Therapeutic gambles outpace conventional ethical norms and can lead to more formalized experimentation—if not here, then elsewhere. In June 2005, the journal *Circulation* published the results of a Pfizer-sponsored study showing that sildenafil had helped children with pulmonary hypertension walk farther and breathe more easily. That year, the FDA approved the drug for the alleviation of PAH symptoms. Beyond the medical and commercial value created by such research, what, other than the immediacy of trial treatment, is owed its subjects?

As I conducted my fieldwork, engaging actors in the global clinical trials industry—businesspeople such as Evan and CRO professionals such as Dr. Coons—and then interpreting and juxtaposing their narratives, I was struck by how freely they could move between the different tiers of health care, seeming as comfortable with patient-volunteers as with private-practice physicians, with corporate managers as with national regulators and local researchers. They conveyed an intimate familiarity with the needs of different medical professionals and patients and, at the same time, broke molds and fostered productive zones where medicine and profit could mix. One small patient recruitment firm, for instance, was founded and continues to be directed by a medically well-connected intensive care nurse. The founder of a small CRO in Eastern Europe had no medical credentials but had an M.B.A. Some were physicians trained at prestigious medical schools in the United States and abroad, who had moved from academic medicine to the industry and to contract research work, or had left powerful positions in government regulatory agencies to become consultants to the industry. Some with M.D./Ph.D.'s had left public health work for jobs in the pharmaceutical industry and then jumped into the trials business. The field was open. They spoke of their expertise as being "cobbled together" and of "writing their own job descriptions." A new workforce had emerged whose purpose was to recruit not only patients but also medical, academic, and governmental actors, bringing them into the permeable fold of the clinical research industry and into profitable relations with each other.

We will meet more of these pragmatic entrepreneurs throughout the book, but now I shift attention to some of the scientists-turned-businessmen who founded the global trials industry in the 1970s. By mastering novel regulatory demands, they carved out independent business niches for themselves. They found ways to institute the testing that was required for an expanding pharmaceutical industry. As these self-made experts mined new opportunities, they turned subcontracting into an important extension of industrial drug development, both at home and abroad. They are not the scientific discoverers of drugs per se, but as they invent the means to move new drugs from bench to bedside, they become "translational scientists" in their own right, helping to transform scientific discoveries into marketable applications. In what follows, I show how the practices of these commercial- and regulatory-savvy actors shape the science and ethics of an evolving global experimentality.

Drug-Development Services

Managers of several contract research organizations urged me to contact Dr. Hein Besselaar, widely regarded as the founder of the clinical-research outsourcing industry. "He knows the history of CROs like no one else," one of his business colleagues told me. A Dutch-born physician, Dr. Besselaar had worked at the National Institutes of Health and in the pharmaceutical industry before becoming, in the mid-1970s, one of the first to establish a drug-development services company. People had cautioned me that Dr. Besselaar traveled widely and was not easy to reach. I persisted for several months, and in October 2003 he returned my call. I told him about my anthropological background and what my study was about. Most historical analysis of clinical research in the twentieth century has focused on government-sponsored research, I said, and I want to illuminate the parallel yet often elusive role of the industry in this history. I said I had specific queries but would be happy if he could guide our conversation in a way he thought was appropriate. "Yes, let's schedule a meeting," I was glad to hear him respond.

After giving me specific directions to his office, Dr. Besselaar told me, "You'll see the huge glass tower over my company." His secretary greeted me and, bringing me to a rather tidy room with floral print wall hangings and lacy curtains, asked me to wait. This traditional decorative style gave very little hint of the legendary man I had heard so much about. Dr. Besselaar, whose career spanned major evolutionary stages in pharmaceutical medicine, was also an avid art connoisseur. He had assembled "a distinguished collection of nineteenth-century Dutch Master paintings. He was a jazz pianist and an avid wine collector. He also enjoyed architecture, design, automobiles, and golf."[5] I was told that he lived in the United States half the year; "otherwise he lived in Bermuda." Ecologically minded, he financially supported a major biological research station there.

Dr. Besselaar was a much-admired, stalwart man whose presence, with his piercing gaze, heavily accented English, and imposing but also somewhat modest manner, was vividly impressive. As we sat down on beige sofas separated by a glass coffee table, it struck me that this was the room of a man who normally was quite literally someplace else. I told him that I wanted to collect his account of the history of outsourced clinical trials management— what brought him to it, what kind of expertise he had developed, and, more generally, how government regulation in drug development affected his work and the conduct of global clinical trials over time. He told me had only one hour, which ended up stretching to a few hours more.

First, Dr. Besselaar wanted to know the difference between my work and journalism. He told me that he had had a bad experience with a journalist, who had "twisted his words" to fit a preconceived line of argument. Anthropologists, on the other hand, take pride in refraining from such an approach. I explained to him that both journalists and anthropologists engage contemporary problems, but methodologically anthropologists strive to gain an insider's perspective and to understand actors on their own terms—ideally, to situate their practices in a broader historical and comparative light. This takes time, charting networks, entering into the perspectives of multiple actors and juxtaposing their diverse viewpoints and stakes. I knew that his specific craft, knowledge, and vision had shaped the modus operandi of contract research, and I felt I needed his account to put the puzzle together. He was glad to help, he said.[6]

"This is going to be a combination of my personal history as well as the history of the contract research industry," he began. "So if I talk a little too much about my personal history, you just eliminate that from whatever you plan to do." Born in Rotterdam in 1935, Dr. Besselaar received his doctorate in internal medicine from the University of Leiden Medical School and became the university's chief resident in internal medicine. He portrayed his training in unpretentious terms and periodically drew sharp distinctions between his work and the work of "academic drug science":

> By 1961, I got interested in how drugs were developed mostly by pharmaceutical companies, occasionally by academia, although they have sometimes exaggerated their role in drug development. And I took some extra pharmacology courses. At that point in time, I decided to become an internist, which in Holland was another five years after you do your medical training. So I did that, but I kept an eye on what was happening in drug development in the U.S. Around 1965, work on clinical pharmacology started to creep into the literature.

The 1962 scandal surrounding the drug thalidomide, he continued, had led to sea changes in drug development, and this shaped his educational trajectory: "That was really the situation that set the regulators on their course to make the whole process of drug approval and therefore the regulatory affairs business much more rigid than it was before." Dr. Besselaar deliberately planned his medical training so as to become an expert in drug development within a postthalidomide regulatory era.

Thalidomide is widely known to cause severe birth defects. Synthesized in 1953 by the West German company Chemie Gruenenthal and put on the market in 1957, it was prescribed as a sleeping pill and also used to treat morning sickness in pregnant women. By the early 1960s, it was sold all over the world. It was in 1960 that the Richardson-Merrell pharmaceutical company submitted an application to the FDA to market the drug in the United States. Random patient testimonials claimed that the drug (like other then-fashionable remedies for nervousness) promoted a good night's rest, but thalidomide had not been thoroughly tested in pregnant animals and women prior to marketing. Soon, reports of infants with incomplete hands or feet sprouting from bodily trunks, and these abnormalities' connection with thalidomide, were published in major medical journals. Some ten thousand children in forty-six countries were found to have been born with thalidomide-induced deformities.[7]

The thalidomide crisis served as a wake-up call, alerting the government to the drug industry's lax testing standards and opening up what Dr. Besselaar characterized as "the regulatory affairs business." Prior to 1962, the drug industry had been free to test new compounds "on the basis of whatever pharmacologic and toxicologic data seemed sufficient," wrote William Wardell and Louis Lasagna (1975:16)—key actors in shaping debates over drug regulation in the United States. Regulations in drug testing, the authors pointed out, varied by country. Some drugs received extensive preclinical workup, while others underwent "the skimpiest of testing in animals" (ibid.). In 1959, for example, the Beacham company launched a new antibiotic based on only two weeks of toxicity tests. At that time, they wrote, when industry approached physicians to perform clinical studies, most participating doctors did not ask to see safety data.

The United States was largely spared the brunt of the thalidomide disaster, partly owing to the diligence of Canadian-born Frances Kelsey, trained in medicine and pharmacology, who had been appointed as medical officer at the FDA in 1960. The application that Richardson-Merrell submitted for regulatory approval of thalidomide fell into Kelsey's hands; in fact, it was her first application review. When Kelsey required more safety data, the company resisted. Finally, it withdrew its application in March 1962, when news of thalidomide's toxicity became widely reported.

Public scrutiny of thalidomide came at just the right time for Senator Estes Kefauver, chair of the Senate Subcommittee on Antitrust and Monopoly, who had been holding hearings about the production of new drugs of dubious efficacy and high drug prices. The hearings had been only mildly successful, and the senator seized the thalidomide crisis as an opportunity to push for greater industry regulation. The 1962 Kefauver-Harris Amendments to the Federal Food, Drug, and Cosmetic Act authorized the FDA to review drug applications not only in terms of their safety, a mandate it had held since 1938, but now explicitly for efficacy as well.[8] The United States became the first country to institute such a proof-of-efficacy requirement in law. While the Kefauver hearings did little to curb either high drug pricing or the industry's penchant for me-too drugs, they did bring about a major overhaul of regulatory practice by establishing the efficacy rule for new treatments (with a focus on randomization and double-blinding and requiring premarket approval of all new drug claims).[9] Controlled clinical trials were now a requirement in proving drug effectiveness and a condition for regulatory approval of a new drug. While it had been in development prior to 1962, clinical pharmacology—the study of drugs in healthy volunteers and patients—was now set in law. It was this new field of "regulatory science" that captured the young Besselaar's interests and decisively altered the institutional ecology of drug development.[10]

A tightly regulated approach to testing experimental compounds resolved some problems but also introduced new ones for drug makers. Who would become its expert? Dr. Besselaar recounted: "People felt that the average physician did not know enough about drugs, and that there was room for a new specialty for people with a medical degree focusing on mechanisms: how drugs worked, what drugs did to the body, and what the body did to drugs. It had much to do with pharmacokinetics, with all the parts of pharmacokinetics: with absorption of drugs, with distribution of drugs, etc., and its impetus came particularly from the U.K. and the U.S." Dr. Besselaar described the new clinical trials approach "as a sort of a menu that you had to work your way through." He organized his postgraduate medical studies to become a clinical trials expert: "Some people really did not know what they were talking about when they said, 'Well, we have a molecule here and we want to investigate that.'"

In 1967, a Merck International Fellowship in Clinical Pharmacology and Medicine brought the young Besselaar to the Experimental Therapeutics Division of the National Institutes of Health in Bethesda, Maryland. "Either because I had the right sponsors or because I was lucky, I got one of those fellowships." He conducted basic laboratory research and simultaneously completed a doctorate in pharmacology at George Washington University. Dr. Besselaar said this diverse training afforded a "marvelous combination" of basic laboratory and clinical research, along with a fundamental knowledge of the statistical aspects of biology.

After obtaining his Ph.D. in 1971, he returned to Holland to fulfill academic and financial obligations linked to the fellowship. "I was a little disappointed in what little happened in the time I had been away. There hadn't been much growth in interest in clinical pharmacology. There were jobs available but not in the exact niche in which I wanted to work." After paying off his debts to the university, he started to explore opportunities in the

United States. "And that was not difficult, because there were many universities that wanted to start clinical pharmacology departments. And since I had the right training and came from the right places, I was a candidate and was offered a number of these positions." He was invited by a fellow Dutchmen, "a social friend of ours, the president of Merck," to launch a new clinical pharmacology division with responsibility for domestic and international early-phase drug development. Dr. Besselaar spent four and half years outfitting the company's drug-testing capabilities in Western Europe, as well as in the United States. He set up studies with investigators and monitored them on site. "So I ended up being responsible for Phase 1 trials for dosaging and safety and early Phase 2 trials for safety and efficacy, on a worldwide basis."

It was not until 1970, eight years after the passage of the Kefauver-Harris Act, that the FDA published regulations that actually defined what "adequate and well-controlled investigations, including clinical investigations," meant. It specified that investigators should include a randomly assigned control group and "use appropriate statistical methods" to allow a "quantitative evaluation" of treatment effects. Dr. Besselaar recalled these times as overly bureaucratic and uncertain. He claimed that most academic scientists were ill prepared to design and carry out trials in accordance with the new rules. FDA drug reviewers, also overwhelmed with new tasks, lacked the technical expertise to review the quality of new drug applications. The antagonism of his retrospective account bespeaks a new competitive arena that emerged in tandem with regulatory science. By the early 1970s, all the frustration came to a head when pharmaceutical industrialists began blaming the government's regulations for the so-called drug lag (1972). This term was coined by two of Dr. Besselaar's colleagues, Drs. William Wardell and Louis Lasagna, who analyzed differences in drug regulatory policy in the United States, the United Kingdom, and other European countries. They claimed that the new regulations had had a stifling effect on the U.S. pharmaceutical industry's rate of innovation and had obstructed the public's timely access to lifesaving drugs. They campaigned for postmarketing safety surveillance of new drugs and opposed the "premarket restrictions" of the new regulations.[11]

The restrictions that these authors spoke of were prohibitive in other senses. Since its 1938 authorization to review the safety and composition of new drugs, the FDA has taken an "informational approach" to defining a new drug's risk and benefits; technically speaking, it regulates drug labeling, not drugs per se or medical practice (Marks 2008:3). In doing so, it has neatly demarcated its authority from other realms, namely, the realms of prescription. In the regulatory approval process, all drug firms have to show is that their drugs are safe for use "under the conditions prescribed, recommended or suggested" in the labeling (ibid.). For drug approval purposes, and until very recently, what has been regulated is the initial testing of a new drug over relatively short periods of time. It is the "displacement" of the experiment onto the nonregulated and autonomous terrains of drug prescription that has become the real worry from a safety perspective. I will contemplate the significance of this displacement for trial offshoring—specifically, of how my CRO interlocutors evaluate the risks and benefits of globalizing trials from a safety perspective. But it is enough to say here that the risk-benefit approach that characterizes modern drug regulation also provided a venue for experimentality in its many forms (as a form of new capital and as a potentially dangerous blurring of lines between the subjects of drug research and real patients and consumers).[12]

The 1962 drug amendments also instituted an instrumental definition of humans taking part in research. From a regulatory point of view, human subjects were now taken as means to an end; they had to be chosen carefully to ensure attainment of the required evidence of safety and efficacy. Drug developers complained, for example, that the new regulations set overly strict rules for patient participation (otherwise known as "inclusion and exclusion criteria") in studies. These criteria include such factors as severity of disease, duration of disease, age, sex, and the use of drugs or therapy other than the experimental drug (so-called concomitant therapies). As Dr. Besselaar put it, the goal was to achieve uniformity of study subjects, "to make sure that the patient population was as uniform as possible [particularly in Phase 3 studies]." Such uniformity supposedly ensured more meaningful, and more valid, comparisons between treatment and control groups. But for Dr. Besselaar and others, these new demands only made drug development more difficult. The drug industry, he said, had to find ways of dealing with such regulatory-made "problems." Consultants like him would mine the gap between regulation and drug development needs. They would provide investigators, compliance services fulfilling human subjects protection mandates, expertise in clinical trials management, as well as an increasingly difficult-to-find right patient:

> We in the industry had a joke: If you take a protocol and follow it to the letter of each inclusion and exclusion criterion for accruing patients, you will find only one patient in the world, and that one patient will say, "I don't want to be part of a clinical trial." So that was sort of

a funny way of letting the FDA know that they were basically on the wrong track. You now had to throw out so many people that eventually, tongue in cheek, you would not find anyone. And that became known as the Law of Lasagna.

Louis Lasagna was a "very, very close friend of mine," Dr. Besselaar added. Dr. Lasagna passed away in 2003 at the age of eighty, just a few weeks before I spoke to Dr. Besselaar. A trained physician and lifelong academic, the New York–born Dr. Lasagna was a pioneer in clinical pharmacology, establishing one of the first clinical pharmacology departments (at Johns Hopkins University). He later cofounded the Center for the Study of Drug Development at the University of Rochester with Dr. William Wardell, who had come to the United States as a Merck International Fellow in Clinical Pharmacology and Medicine. In 1984, the center moved to Tufts University. Dr. Lasagna played a key role in the Kefauver hearings and in establishing controlled trials as the basis for the FDA's drug efficacy standards. Like Dr. Besselaar, he was highly sensitive to the practical uncertainties that the new architecture of drug development introduced.

Some of his specific insights are captured in the well-known "Law of Lasagna" that Dr. Besselaar alluded to during our discussion. In any trial, so says the law, investigators will overestimate the number of patients that can be obtained for the study—recruitment always falls short of expectation. Overly strict inclusion criteria often do not reflect the prevalence of the disorder on which a trial's sample size calculations are based. Moreover, recruitment of eligible patients might also be biased by "physician and patient motivation" (Huibers et al. 2004:213). While Lasagna, the academic, focused on the potential for miscalculations and misfires in patient recruitment, Dr. Besselaar built on his drug industry experience in international early-phase trials and began to manage and monitor Phase 2 and much larger Phase 3 trials.

In those early days, recalls Dr. Besselaar, "I had developed a knack for the architecture of drug development. Where you can really make a difference is in how Phase 1, 2, and 3 studies complement and fit into each other. You often do forty or fifty different kinds of studies in order to produce the evidence needed to support one drug application." As a one-man consultant to the pharmaceutical industry, he said, "I could help a lot from a theoretical point of view, showing companies the best way to develop the drug." An instrumental approach to human subjects took form under the new regulatory regime, and Dr. Besselaar advanced a new enterprise around this instrumentalism.

For example, I would say the first study should be in ten patients or maybe we should have ten different Phase 1 studies, followed by five different Phase 2 studies, and then seven different Phase 3 studies. I would also say these are the drugs you have to compare the experimental drug to, and these are the dosages of the drugs you have to compare them with . . . these are the summary protocols as to what kinds of patients you've got to put into the trial. And all this turned out to be an assumption that worked.

It worked, said Dr. Besselaar, but not with "the established pharmaceutical companies, because they would all say, 'Oh, we know all that,' even if they didn't." Instead, it worked, "fortunately," with a couple of big companies that wanted to diversify and venture into pharmaceuticals. "And one of those was Procter & Gamble." Dr. Besselaar became a consultant to this multiproduct company, helping to identify drugs that had potential for human development. This consulting work was the beginning of the company that "I immodestly called G. H. Besselaar Associates. There were no associates in the beginning, but after about two years, there were probably about ten of us. And we also started to execute international trials instead of just being consultants."

From Vulnerable to Professional Subjects

The FDA's stricter research oversight in the wake of the thalidomide crisis, Dr. Besselaar told me, "made it much more difficult to initiate research in the United States." This was particularly true for Phase 1 studies: "You had to file an investigational new drug [IND] application with the FDA. They weren't very fast in coming back to you with questions. And if there were questions, it took time for us to reach an agreement on [the design of the] protocol. In some countries in Western Europe—Eastern Europe wasn't accessible to us yet—study start-up was much quicker. Thus a lot of the Phase 1 and even early Phase 2 research crossed the Atlantic Ocean, from the U.S. to Europe."

One point of origin for this movement of early phase trials (for toxicity studies that are called "nontherapeutic") dates back to the early 1970s, when state-supported institutions (prisons and mental hospitals, for example), which had provided access to volunteers and controlled conditions for research, ceased to be easily accessible. Prison environments possessed many desirable features for research (particularly behavioral research). The population was more or less stable, and life was "subject to few variations"

(Annas, Glantz, and Katz 1977:103). Clinical research among prisoners was accepted practice during the first half of the twentieth century and flourished in the 1950s and 1960s. Back then, debating its ethics was not high on political and public agendas (Hoffman 2000). "In the old days," Dr. Besselaar told me, "one could use prison populations for Phase 1 [drug toxicity] studies. All that changed very soon after I entered the industry."

Companies queued up for prison populations. Some even acquired exclusive rights to construct research facilities adjoining or very near prisons. Upjohn and Parke-Davis, for example, ran laboratories and had monitoring rooms and hospital beds in a research center built next to Michigan's Jackson State Prison. After 1972, research on prisoners—"difficult, if not impossible, to duplicate elsewhere"—came under intensely negative public scrutiny (Mitford 1973:62). Social critic Jessica Mitford penned an in-depth and wrenching report called "Experiments behind Bars," which described the extent of activity and identified the stakeholders involved in research on prisoners. Drug companies, she wrote, operated through private physicians who could access prisoners. Prison wardens and correctional facility physicians acted as brokers, allowing company representatives to canvass their prisoner populations for eligible volunteers. Companies paid correctional officers and physicians directly. Contracts were verbal. Prisoners, while not allowed to earn money, often received nominal rewards for their involvement. Medical school researchers were enrolled to conduct prison research. In one case, academic researchers created a nonprofit organization through which payments for this prison-related research could be channeled (ibid.:70).

The debate over whether prisoners were free to participate or coerced into research was not easily settled.[13] Neither was the issue of what consequences for drug development would stem from the outlawing of nontherapeutic research (Phase 1 studies, for example) on prisoners. Dr. Besselaar recalled that the critics of such research focused on "free will" but did not necessarily account for some of the benefits volunteers enjoyed for signing up for a trial. "They did get other advantages. They didn't have to be on the chain gang; they probably got more regular food. They were not allowed to get paid but . . . they were on their bed waiting for the next blood stick. For a lot of people that was attractive."

During our conversation, Dr. Besselaar did not convey any sense of engagement with the heated debates over the ethics of human research that marked the early seventies, when the great ethical scandals came to light. The most prominent of these, the Tuskegee syphilis experiment, catalyzed the new governance of research conduct as well as the rise of modern bioethics. The mainstreaming of trials and their internationalization seem to have fully occupied Dr. Besselaar's attention. He anticipated the industry's need for expertise and reliable business partners in facilitating trials elsewhere. This early offshoring of trials provided a different context altogether from which he might engage (or disengage from) these national debates.

I remarked to Dr. Besselaar that Louis Lasagna, for example, had defended the value of using prisoners as research subjects on scientific grounds (1977). The control over inmates' daily lives, habits, medicinal intake, and food consumption—in contrast to the more chaotic and difficult-to-monitor outside world—would have helped researchers fulfill the new mandates for patient uniformity much more proficiently. This argument echoed earlier ones over the scientific "merits" of using prisoner volunteers in gonorrhea studies during World War II. While the results of that research were "meager," they convinced organizers that "[r]esearch on humans worth doing was worth doing well" (Marks 1997:105). In responding, Dr. Besselaar did not directly address Lasagna's argument but, rather, mentioned prisoners' letters, published in major medical journals, stating their desire to be guinea pigs. "But the weakness of their argument," he said, "was that you never knew how research was done in every location. In the best locations, it was probably handled quite well, but we don't have any idea of how it was handled everywhere." Dr. Besselaar declined to take sides in this debate over whether prisoner research was scientifically superior or operationally expedient. He was, instead, articulating an alternative route toward new investigators and research subjects. "I was on the side of the people who said you really have to find a patient population that is more informed, that has a true free will, and that can walk away from the research at any moment they want to, which in a prison setting was not so easy." He paused and finished his train of thought, "And we really went after what we called normal volunteers."

But this was easier said than done. Initially, "drifters" in need of money enlisted, he said, but they were inappropriate from the start: "A lot of them had to be excluded because they were alcoholics or drug addicts. They were not very dependable." Dr. Besselaar's task was to find "more reliable" subject populations, particularly for Phase 1 studies. Site selection for a clinical trial necessarily takes into consideration the choice to use certain groups over others. "My own preference is to work with medical students. They are the best informed and they have proven that they have an I.Q. that makes them capable of understanding a piece of paper stating the pros and cons [of the research] and that talks about side effects. They can walk out of it at any point in time if they so desire. And they ask a thousand and one questions about it, which is good." In this discourse, the ideal experimental subject is a capable subject as opposed to the vulnerable subject who had come under strict regulatory protection. Dr. Besselaar and everyone else in the industry would have to "make do" with "more professional" subjects. As federal regulators made legal distinctions between restricted research populations and unrestricted free agents of research, the clinical trials industry would thrive in identifying the latter. Besselaar's retrospection, as partial as it is, provides an account of a risk-benefit approach to research populations as it evolved internationally, and of how experimentality became an industrialized field in its own right.

⚜

As historians of science and medicine have amply documented, experimental subjects have been disproportionately and routinely drawn from disadvantaged or marginalized groups. Many have participated in research without full knowledge and consent. Their participation in experiments has often been directly linked to poverty or to an institutionalized lack of rights. The diseased condition that becomes the pretext for their involvement has often been shaped by institutional neglect or by research conditions themselves, or by some combination of the two. Precisely such a combination occurred in the notorious Willowbrook hepatitis study.[14]

For fourteen years, starting in 1956, government-funded researchers infected behaviorally impaired children institutionalized at the Willowbrook State School in New York with the hepatitis A virus, allowing researchers to observe the natural course of infectious hepatitis. Investigators defended their actions by stating that the vast majority of the children they injected would have acquired the disease anyway during their stay at Willowbrook. They said that the experiment posed no additional risks because the context inflicted more damage than they would inflict through "mere" research. As a matter of historical record, hepatitis outbreaks had occurred at Willowbrook prior to the experiment. Infamously, researchers suggested that it would be *better* for the children to be infected under controlled conditions of research.

Experimentality of this kind, in which claims of a damage-inflicting context could trump ethics was, arguably, essential to the undertaking. Similarly, in 1963, researchers injected live cancer cells into individuals with disabling chronic diseases who were patients at New York City's Jewish Chronic Disease Hospital. The scientists wanted to understand the nature of the human transplant rejection process. They felt that obtaining documented consent was not necessary because these patients were subjected to many injurious medical practices anyway.

The Tuskegee syphilis experiment has been called the longest nontherapeutic experiment on human beings in medical history (Jones 1981 [1993]). From 1932 to 1972, nineteen researchers of the U.S. Public Health Service observed four hundred black sharecroppers in Macon County and Tuskegee, Alabama, monitoring the natural course of these men's advanced untreated syphilis. Two hundred disease-free men acted as controls. Penicillin, discovered in the late 1940s to be an appropriate treatment for syphilis, could have saved many of these subjects' lives, but it was denied.[15]

Disclosures of research abuse spurred Congress to pass the 1974 National Research Act. This act called for the establishment of institutional review boards to evaluate the ethical conduct of research. It also authorized the formation of the National Commission for the Protection of Human Subjects of Biomedical and Behavioral Research.[16] The commission was asked to identify basic ethical principles that should underlie research involving human subjects and to develop guidelines for their protection that would be codified in law. The commission was to consider the boundaries between biomedical and behavioral research and routine medical practice; risk-benefit criteria in the determination of the appropriateness of human subjects research and appropriate guidelines for the selection of subjects; and the nature and definition of informed consent in various research contexts.[17]

The commission deliberated over the conditions of research among vulnerable research subjects such as children, prisoners, pregnant women, and mentally disabled persons. These deliberations over who should be excluded from participation in research were strongly shaped by the politics of the time. In the wake of the 1973 Supreme Court's decision in *Roe v. Wade*, not surprisingly, the commission first dealt with the use of aborted fetuses in clinical research. In the coming years, "women of childbearing age [were] barred from most clinical research, either legislatively or through manufacturers' fear of litigation" (Brada 2004:8).

In 1975, commission members visited the Jackson State Prison in Michigan. They learned of the active markets afforded by the presence of pharmaceutical investigators and competition among prisoners for the chance of taking part in the drug research projects. As the commissioners started working on ethical guidelines that would strike "a good, right, and just balance between all the different moral claims arising within the context of research involving human subjects from one group to another," they reportedly started to rethink their "paternalistic" conceptions of prisoners as being vulnerable and coerced (Toulmin 1987:606). The prisoners were apparently not as vulnerable as the commissioners had initially thought. But just before the commission was ready to make its recommendation to the Department of Health, Education and Welfare (HEW)—in fact, a recommendation that prisons be kept open for research under certain conditions (ibid.)—the wall came crashing down. The U.S. Bureau of Prisons—in what philosopher Stephen Toulmin interprets as an apparent move to absolve itself from future liability and to brashly display its own ability to self-regulate—"changed its policies, so as to exclude effectively all research by drug companies and other outside agencies from federal prisons" (ibid.). In 1978, HEW followed suit and formally decided to dramatically limit federally funded research involving prisoners (in 1979, HEW became the Department of Health and Human Services).

That year, the commission issued the report *Ethical Principles and Guidelines for the Protection of Human Subjects of Research*, known as *The Belmont Report*. The report summarized ethical principles that form the core of the Department of Health and Human Services (HHS) human subjects protection regulations. Respect for persons and individual autonomy were to be assured by informed consent procedures. Beneficence should be systematically assessed, and research should maximize possible benefits and minimize possible harms. The principle of justice was affirmed: the benefits and risks of research should be distributed through fair procedures. These guidelines revised and expanded federal regulation.[18] The so-called Common Rule establishes layers of protection between vulnerable subjects and researchers (in the form of institutional review boards, informed consent, and privacy protections). Prisoners, for example, cannot be subjects of non-therapeutic trials, nor can they be used as a population of convenience.

The Belmont Report created a categorical distinction between a person who is capable of self-determination and one who is not, and it introduced a particular notion of the morally competent self: "Some persons are in need of extensive protection, even to the point of excluding them from activities which may harm them." These vulnerable populations must be excluded from research for their own protection. By contrast, "other persons require little protection beyond making sure they undertake activities freely and with awareness of possible adverse consequences. The extent of protection afforded should depend upon the risk of harm and the likelihood of benefit." The report left open the possibility of including (or further excluding) certain populations depending on circumstance. "The judgment that any individual lacks autonomy should be periodically reevaluated and will vary in different situations."[19]

Indeed, a myriad of media events and legislative decisions led to the constitution of this consent-based regulatory model for biomedical and behavioral research. So long as an investigator could document that his or her subjects could deliberate about personal goals and act "under the direction of such deliberation," it was ultimately up to the subjects themselves to judge the acceptability of the risks they took. No external agency would be in a position to declare their activities—or their deliberations—"outside" legal requirements.[20] This privatized and highly individualized risk-benefit approach underwrites the global clinical trial.

In Dr. Besselaar's account, the clinical research enterprise is in a symbiotic relationship with state regulation, and internationalization affords a new revenue stream. This entangled history of regulation and outsourcing and offshoring provides a different standpoint from which to assess the evolution of research ethics in the United States. The government's rule making created logistical barriers that, in turn, "displaced" research elsewhere and enabled a whole new chapter in globalized research.[21] I probed specifically how the new research regulations of the 1970s affected his work. Again, the answer was pragmatic and stressed accountability within the new rules, while exploring what could be done in different countries and expanding investigative networks. He particularly addressed Phase 1 testing, as he was still working at Merck in the 1970s:

> It wasn't a problem getting normal volunteers, either in Europe or in the United States. I cannot recall that studies had to be scratched because we couldn't get subjects. And what happened as a result of this was that in Europe some Phase 1 units started to be built. And a number of European entrepreneurs started these units. In England particularly, and sometimes [they were] attached to universities' hospitals and sometimes the research units were purely commercial. Holland, Germany, and France were a bit on the slow side. Italy did not participate. Spain was not a country where you would go. Scandinavia was an excellent region where you would go, particularly Sweden, where you would go for Phase 1 research.

In answer to my question, "Why Sweden?" he responded, succinctly, that the "infrastructure was excellent." By that he meant, among other things, that a formalized ethical review process was in place: "There, the ethical side of research received a lot of attention. Sweden was one of the first countries to start ethical review committees, and they functioned very well," which meant that companies could initiate trials more quickly. Sweden also had scientific experts in high bureaucratic positions who could judge the validity of protocols. After building up the capabilities of Phase 1 and early Phase 2 research in Europe, Dr. Besselaar also became responsible for these activities in the United States and for "making contacts with thousands of investigators who do all phases of testing worldwide."

In 1981, when the Department of Health and Human Services and the Food and Drug Administration issued regulations based on *The Belmont Report,* drug companies, according to Besselaar's time line, had already shifted some of their Phase 1 work to other countries. Dr. Besselaar was being offered many jobs like the one he had at Merck, but they all "looked exactly the same." He wanted to do something new. He left the pharmaceutical industry and founded his own research firm. "'Gentlemen,' we said, 'we are available to execute your study.'"

The primary goal of contract research organizations, he told me, is "to get drugs approved. The other one is to kill bad drugs as quickly as possible, because if we kill them quickly, companies don't have to spend a tremendous amount of money. [The sponsors] can use it on something else that could have a chance." Getting drugs approved and killing drugs quickly require different kinds of experts and evidence-gathering strategies. In what follows, I explore the opportunities the pharmaceutical boom of the 1980s and 1990s created for clinical research and how this new enterprise evolved in tandem with a changing environment of decision making over ethical mandates and legal norms.

The Pharmaceutical Boom and Everyday Research

As the foregoing brief foray into the history of industry-sponsored research through the 1970s suggests, drugs increasingly came to be tested in "general populations" in the United States and Western Europe, where the major pharmaceutical markets were. Trials took place mostly in academic medical settings. Dr. Besselaar recalled dealing with academic investigators who were interested in the research and not necessarily the money. "Things were very straightforward," he told me, adding that these were the "good old days."

> Financial negotiations were always very brief. I asked the investigator if he knew twenty subjects. If he said yes, I would ask him to calculate his time and the time of his study coordinator and nurse, how much laboratory work was involved, and what all that was going to cost. 'Come back to us with a cost per patient.' And after he came back, we

would say yes or no. Many of the people involved did it not on the basis of the money, but based on their interest in the drug. So those were the good days, those were the easy days, compared to where we are today, which is a different story altogether.

A pharmaceutical boom was imminent. "The watershed year was 1980. Before then, it was a good business, but afterward, it was a stupendous one. From 1960 to 1980, prescription drug sales were fairly static as a percent of US gross domestic product, but from 1980 to 2000, they tripled. They now stand at more than $200 billion a year" (Angell 2004). This "bonanza" was enabled by a series of business-friendly legislative decisions. The 1980 University and Small Business Patent Procedures Act, also known as the Bayh-Dole Act, granted academic institutions and small firms the power to patent discoveries derived from research sponsored by the National Institutes of Health and then to grant licensing rights to the pharmaceutical industry. It encouraged collaboration between academic researchers and corporations and fostered biotechnology industry growth. Four years later, Congress passed the Drug Price Competition and Patent Term Restoration Act (the Hatch-Waxman Act), promoting the entrance of generics into the market but lengthening the patent life for brand-name drugs. The industry re-tooled some of the act's provisions and found legal loopholes to extend patents far longer than anticipated, resulting in a significant source of income. "Since the act was passed, brand-name drug companies routinely file not just one patent on their drugs but a series of them spread throughout the life of the first patent. These secondary patents are on every conceivable attribute—never mind usefulness, novelty, or non-obviousness" (Relman and Angell 2002:36).

Drug makers could employ several strategies to extend the life of medications whose patents were set to expire. They could test one medication in combination with another—a blood pressure drug with a cholesterol drug, for example, or an antipsychotic drug with an antidepressant—to create "dual use" drugs.[22] They could also search for new uses for already approved drugs or create successor versions of them. By 1994, for example, "hundreds of studies on the relative merits" of similar antacid products were under way (Goozner 2004:219). Under FDA rules, in most circumstances, drug makers do not have to compare their drugs with the best standard of care or with existing drugs treating the same condition, but with a placebo. The "me-too" drugs that often result revitalized the pharmaceutical pipeline. Fast-forward a decade later, they remain the major output of the industry. Of the 93 drugs approved in 2006, 73 were me-too drugs. As one CRO scientist said to me, "Drugs on the market are so similar, pharma companies want to find very small differences that will show that their drug is superior, somehow. But in order to prove that one small aspect, you need a very, very select patient population, and that's why trials are getting more complicated." He will explain what he means by "more complicated" in chapter 3. "If you have a totally new drug, it is much easier to prove that it works or that it has fewer side effects."

By the 1980s, the industry was also entering the era of the megatrial, marked by large-scale, statistically powered multicentered trials that enrolled and sampled significantly larger numbers of people. The therapeutic benefits of new drugs were becoming less pronounced, and the benefits that were too modest to measure in small trials could be magnified in larger ones. Trials grew in scope and complexity. By the mid-1980s, drug firms—pressed to contain costs and deal with their own operational limits—started outsourcing data management and statistical analysis functions as well as traditionally internal functions such as laboratory and clinical research operations (Winter and Baguley 2006:2; Rettig 2000:134). Biotechnology firms also outsourced to augment capacities and resources that they lacked internally.

The reorganization of the pharmaceutical industry and the emergence of biotech occasioned new business opportunities for independent-minded entrepreneurs: "Most of the individuals who started CROs were opportunistic. They thought there are peaks and valleys of demand, that is, outside help that companies wouldn't want to make permanent—and therein lay a business opportunity," Rob Gordon, the CEO of Tem/po, told me. "Most CROs started as a cottage industry, very small, out of garages with a few computers, scientists, people who came out of pharma and said, 'I can take on some of this data management work or trial monitoring on a contract basis,' and ran at a small scale probably until the mid-1990s. These were people who came out of pharma with experience, but initially the industry did not trust them with anything large or complicated." Gordon (who had worked in drug firms most of his professional life) said drug firms initially viewed CROs as "sort of adjunct to the labor force that we had internally."

As CROs helped firms to transcend the limits of their capacity, they began offering "fields of expertise that the industry chose not to create," as one founder of a leading global contract research organization told me in a conversation in 2003. A medically trained pharmaceutical expert, he developed the international research programs of several major pharmaceutical companies into the 1980s. This professional made a name for himself in the fiercely competitive "antacid wars," as he was involved in the research program for one of the largest-selling drugs of its time. His efforts helped save the manufacturer from decreasing profits and upended its chief competitor's sales.

After leaving the pharmaceutical industry in 1985, he began to manage entire drug research programs, first as a private industry consultant, then as founder of a CRO. Companies sought out people like him for time- and expense-reduction strategies, particularly in the second and third phases of trials. "The pharmaceutical companies would come to me and say, 'Our track record of doing clinical development is so poor. Our last beta-blocker,' this is the company talking, 'took ten years from first patient in until approval by the FDA. You say that you can do it in four years, you've got the contract.'"

As for Dr. Besselaar, in 1989, he sold his company to Corning, Inc., a large glass manufacturer eager to venture into the now-profitable field of the life sciences. Corning had already bought the world's largest animal toxicology research laboratory (Hazleton, located in Virginia) and would soon acquire SciCor, a chemical laboratory organization in Indianapolis. Dr. Besselaar managed Corning's drug-development division and extended it to Europe. The company became "the world's biggest contract clinical research organization," he told me. "Corning kept its hands off for the first three years. We did what we wanted to do. We grew from 250 to 1,000 people, and the whole pharmaceutical services group grew to more than 2,000 people." Dr. Besselaar remained on Corning's board until 1996, when the company moved out of pharmaceuticals and into fiber optics. He took his management staff with him and founded an independent contract research organization. Corning's drug-development division also became an independent CRO. By the mid-1990s, CROs went public. As outsourcing as a percentage of total R&D spending by pharmaceutical and biotechnology firms increases, the financial outlook for CROs remains optimistic.[23]

By the early 1990s, research had migrated from academic-based research centers, where it had been principally conducted, to everyday hospital and primary-care settings and for-profit investigative sites. According to Dr. Besselaar, academic hospitals became "too difficult" to negotiate with as new forms of research oversight set in. Beyond that, other drawbacks made these sites "not a good breeding ground for drug studies." While studies for life-threatening diseases generally took place in academic settings, from a practical standpoint "academia did not deliver much in terms of patient numbers, and you had to deal with too many people and administrative layers, from the administration to the researcher to the union staff. And frankly, academics don't want to do the grunt work, the same thing over and over again."

During our conversation, I asked Dr. Besselaar what he thought about the highly publicized deaths of two patients in trials carried out in academic settings a few years earlier.[24] He said he didn't know much about these cases: "I don't follow these things very well, but let me tell you that, in general, there have been far more problems in academic than in nonacademic centers, that's absolutely true." He then focused on what he thought were the more salient problems he had encountered with clinical research in academic institutions. "Many studies are not completed. There is an ethical problem with these studies because you have desperate patients involved. You want to see whether a new treatment might have a chance of working. But if you don't finish the study, you never come up with an answer. So you put people at risk for no answer at all. There are far more of those studies in academia than there are in nonacademic research settings. This happens because academic settings don't have enough patients."

In fact, we have no data on whether more people get injured in academic research settings than at for-profit sites (Caplan 2007). Avoiding the issue of patient injury in his response, Dr. Besselaar suggested that there was a greater price to pay for inefficient drug development. Commercial research moved out of academic settings that, in principle, "don't have enough patients" and "get the very sick patients, the patients who cannot enter into a normal protocol because they have lots of exclusion criteria and so on. It is very difficult for an academic center to really be involved in everyday drug research. They have all tried it because it is a nice sort of income, but it is very hard to do." What he calls "everyday" drug research consisting of "normal" protocols requires larger patient pools and repetitive "grunt work."[25] This everyday research has evolved into a highly profitable enterprise. There are many stakeholders—public and private organizations, investigators, and study participants—bringing multiple and competing interests into the process of negotiating trial contracts, rules of accountability, and degrees of independence from pharmaceutical sponsors and their demands. Relations among all parties tend to be strained; there is no easily accessible and straightforward account of the total phenomenon.

Outlining the structure of sponsorship and recruitment for clinical trials in the United States, in cases where an outsourced service provider is involved, is one way to shed further light on how the clinical trials industry is organized. First, there are the pharmaceutical companies or the sponsors who have a new compound to test. Assuming that they wanted to outsource the development of that entity, they would turn to a CRO, which could handle subject recruitment, clinical testing, data management, and drug approval. The CRO might have direct links with investigator sites, or it might act through yet another party, the site management organization (SMO). The latter owns or manages a set of affiliated sites, typically within a defined region, to augment recruitments. At the most basic level of drug testing, there is a principal investigator and an investigative site, which may be a hospital or a hospital ward, a physician group practice, an academic institution, or a for-profit research facility. The principal investigator can contract with the CRO, with the SMO, or directly with the drug's developer. In 2005, CROs handled 71 percent of outsourced research and development (R&D). The SMO share of that market was considerably smaller, only 2 percent. Academic health centers regained some of their lost ground and controlled 26.1 percent of outsourced R&D (CenterWatch 2005:237).

This industry-sponsored research ecology is mutable. Testing sites emerge and disappear. Companies merge and morph into other businesses, creating new chains of value or abandoning old ones. Investigators are constantly honing skills and acquiring new ones—for some physicians, research is a unique opportunity for professional mobility; for others, that opportunity does not pan out in practice. Investigators can shift allegiances and positions, as they, too, "want to get a piece of it all," in the words of Evan, the director of the midwestern branch of Across-the-Globe-Research. To develop a better sense of the ordinary ways in which research evolves, the dilemmas faced and the solutions found, and how these trends affect the business of overseas trials, I undertook a series of interviews with individuals in each tier of the commercial research enterprise.

Consider the work of John Tucker (a pseudonym) the founder of a site management organization based in a major northwestern U.S. city. Tucker is a nurse who worked with trauma and open-heart surgery patients at a large academic hospital. His position gave him the opportunity to interact with many medical specialists and various levels of hospital staff. He knew almost everyone in his hospital, he told me. In the early 1990s, a pharmaceutical firm approached him, and one of his superiors, with a request to facilitate trials in the hospital. Tucker was in a position to deliver. He became a "clinical research coordinator" and began to facilitate patient and investigator recruitments, coordinate research, and negotiate trial contracts between investigators and pharmaceutical sponsors.

Today, through his company, Mr. Tucker's employees act as liaisons between physicians and local communities and drug sponsors who want to conduct a study. The payoff now is higher. The company manages clinical research in both public and private hospitals. According to its advertising, it has a catalog of motivated doctors and institutions, has access to various patient populations (including ethnic and minority ones), and has a centralized contract negotiation and IRB submission process. Tucker also conducts outreach and public education at community events. It is in his company's interest to heighten public awareness of clinical trials and increase opportunities for subject participation. As he explained, "We are paid for patients enrolled and work completed."

I first met Mr. Tucker at a clinical trials conference. He was happy to tell me about his professional trajectory. His transition from a nurse to the founder and director of a well-regarded SMO speaks of a self-made expertise. It is also a story about the evolution of new infrastructural arrangements in the facilitation and management of commercialized clinical trials. Mr. Tucker presented his story as one of instant success. His first clinical trial involved a longitudinal study of cardiac patients. On the basis of that study, he said, "I raised hundreds of thousands of dollars. I sent all the residents to courses, I bought microscopes and computers, and because we took the money in . . . the only thing that we had to pay was my salary. I mean, literally, we were the highest enrollers for six years on this study. We made scads of money."

As his research enterprise within the hospital grew, Tucker and his supervisor decided to market their activities. They gave themselves new titles and "got the cards made up." But in attempting to bring in more industry-sponsored research, he ran into conflict with other administrators. The chairman of a medical department claimed that "we were prostituting the institution by taking this dirty money," said Tucker, "but I don't think it was dirty money." With some administrative maneuvering, they were able to continue their work for a couple of more years—"I was doing a million dollars' worth of research."

Tucker organized a group of people to coordinate meetings among doctors and sponsors. He also began to pool these coordinators and "farm them out" all over the hospital. He had in essence established a freestanding research facility within the hospital. When the hospital president finally took notice, he asked him to return to his previous job. Instead, Tucker moved the business out of the hospital and began working with "community docs." He shared Dr. Besselaar's view that academic hospitals were not preparing themselves "fast enough for what eventually was going to happen": "I used to say to my boss, 'Look at how long it takes for us to get these contracts negotiated and IRB reviews done. The independent people out in the city are getting it done much quicker . . . and that's where I went. To my surprise, after I left, community hospitals started calling us, saying, 'Hey, would you come and set up a research center for us?'" Tucker and colleagues broke traditional occupational molds and traversed different institutions and forms of institutionalized oversight, apparently without too many obstacles. Mobility and risk taking of this sort distinguished the experts of a growing clinical trials industry. They spoke of a time when business gambits paid off and when institutional rules governing academic-industry exchange had not yet fully matured.

By the end of the 1990s, the number of groups of specialized physicians and primary-care doctors who had turned their practices into investigator sites had grown significantly.[26] Tucker's specialty is to facilitate this kind of transformation, providing the staff and expertise necessary for successful implemention of trials. The increased interest in becoming a trial site reflected lowered Medicare reimbursements and changes in the structure of payments by health maintenance organizations (HMOs) and other capitation-based plans. Capitation—as opposed to the traditional fee-for-service model—was introduced in the mid-1990s by HMOs. HMOs pay doctors a fixed sum of money over a specific time period for each patient in their practice, whether they treat that patient seldom or frequently.[27] Doctors turned to clinical trials as a way of recouping some of their diminishing revenues in this new system of payment. But the expected boost in profits often did not materialize.

꒰◇꒱

Members of the contract research organization community I talked to frequently complained that, despite the high development costs[28] of a drug, their pharmaceutical clients have kept payments to CROs "relatively flat," taking advantage of the fact that the CRO market is becoming ever more crowded. From people working in investigative sites, in turn, I heard complaints that payments from pharmaceutical sponsors and CROs were not in step with the inflation of nurses' salaries and the high cost of making sites compliant with current regulatory policies. As one of my informants put it, "The lawyers and the IRBs at all institutions have gotten pickier. The administrative burden and the cost base of labor in investigative sites have gone up enormously, but their reimbursement levels have not."

These economics can have a debilitating effect on the quality of research. They have led, for example, to the pervasive reality of so-called *floater sites*—investigative sites that promise many patients, routinely underbid for contracts, and are not meticulously concerned with achieving standards of safety and compliance (see chapter 1). They make their money and disappear from the clinical trials food chain. "Pharma loves floater sites!" exclaimed a former nurse and now director of a large SMO (like Tucker's) at an industry-sponsored conference in 2004. In 2005, the media reported that a CRO was implicated in a scandal involving a 675-bed Phase 1 and 2 investigative facility in Miami. The site, a converted Holiday Inn, was run by an unlicensed physician. Its research subjects, "many of them poor Hispanic immigrants," were "lured by per-trial payments, enrolled without fully comprehending the risk of injury or death and were enticed to stay in trials in some cases by 'backloading,' in which the largest payments are made near the end of the trial" (Shuchman 2007:1365).

Several trial managers complained about how costly it was to keep up with floater sites and to ensure ethical and safe research. Pharmaceutical sponsors, I was told, do not necessarily want to include coverage of those costs in the contract. The existence of floater sites makes it more difficult for more established investigative sites to get full compensation for expenses such as those associated with study start-up, serious adverse event management, protocol changes, and subject screening failures. Moreover, my informants told me that the proliferation of floater sites has not been matched by an equal expansion of oversight mechanisms, and that they had serious concerns over the reliability of the data these sites produced.

Players in all tiers of the clinical trials ecology invoke the trope of victimization. Pharmaceutical companies say that they are victims of overregulation. CROs and SMOs complain that the pharmaceutical industry underpays and that it does not do enough (read: pay enough) to protect the integrity of the research process and to ensure against possible risks. Medical personnel struggle with the hidden costs of a practice they thought would be less bureaucratic and much more profitable. But all parties keep tinkering with the system and making money. Investigators can use study start-up funds and then not deliver on data. Or they can overbook their investigative sites with clinical trials, which can translate into personnel burnout. One CRO scientist described the problems in these sites in these terms: "Unless the study staff and operations are run like sweatshops, there's no economic profitability for the investigator." Given the high demand for certain types of patients, investigators can drop a trial prematurely for a more lucrative one—"Either he is making more money, or I would like to think that he thinks that the new drug will be better for his patient," said a lawyer who negotiates trial contracts for a small pharmaceutical company. Or, if you are a CRO, you can offshore trials, reduce costs, and expand business frontiers elsewhere.

The FDA Office of Compliance suggests that new risks are being introduced with the routinization of commercialized research. The office is receiving an increasing number of complaints filed against investigators.[29] This increase is attributed to protocol violations, falsification of data, informed consent noncompliance, poor adverse event reporting, and poor drug accountability. Individual investigators are typically held responsible for these problems. But these are systemic problems, and the idea of an effective self-regulating clinical research market is far from reality.

Engineering Out Harm

The ethical guidelines for conducting scientific experiments upon humans that have evolved since the establishment of the Nuremberg Code in 1949 emphasize the need for informed and voluntary consent of participants who "should be situated so as to be able to exercise free power of choice."[30] But the elimination of egregious abuses "has tended to highlight more subtle ethical problems" (Iyalomhe and Imomoh 2007:301). In 1968, when the field of bioethics was just beginning to emerge in the United States, the philosopher Hans Jonas expressed grave concerns about the "potentially superior claims" that science could make in the name of progress, claims that might lead individuals to consent to "the ritualized exposure to gratuitous risk of health and life, justified by a presumed greater, social good" (1969: 224).[31] Jonas was skeptical of attempts to present human experimentation as an imperative for progress. "We require a careful clarification," he wrote, "of what the needs, interests, and rights of society are, for society . . . is an abstract and as such is subject to our definition" (ibid.:221).

For Jonas, the idea of informed consent meant something much bigger than its current conventionalized use, which focuses on the protection of personal decisional autonomy.[32] Nor did he have in mind a legal strategy, in the sense of investigators' or nurses' obtaining patient consent and releasing investigators or sponsoring institutions from liability in case of adverse effects or negligence. For him, consent was an empirical capacity and a deliberative intelligence about the purpose and value of knowledge and a force working against the dangers of the "unknown in our problem," or what constitutes "the so-called common or public good." Without a political-economic and social understanding that could justify choice, the scope of informed consent remains limited at best. Speaking directly with some of the architects and agents of the decentralization and expansion of commercial research, one grasps the concrete limits of informed consent in its legal, contractual, and doctrinal form.

Now in his mid-sixties, an amicable and soft-spoken CRO scientist I call Dr. Everett Keel is an industry expert whom Rob Gordon, then Tem/po's CEO, referred me to regarding all questions of ethics. I met and spoke with him several times over the years. Dr. Keel obtained his M.D. and a Ph.D. in biostatistics at a prestigious medical school in the United States. He had worked for several large pharmaceutical firms for most of his professional life before joining Tem/po in 1997. When I had asked him in 2004 to comment on ethics in his enterprise, he referred to the sponsors as the problem. "The ethics is abysmal, the lowest it can get, and I will not mention the sponsors."

In referring to how trials are actually carried out, Dr. Keel identified two ethical registers: "There is the question of human subjects protection during the research process and the question of the generalizability of the data derived from the research process, that is, the basis for predicting drug benefit or harm. These are the two pieces of the equation." He called these ethical registers "trial subjects ethics" and "market ethics." In the first, the idea of vulnerability as drafted in law and regulation is narrow, though he felt patient safety at this level is achievable and patients, by and large, emerge unscathed. He was mostly concerned with market ethics—how the quality of research protocols and competitive environments of research can degrade patient and consumer safety. Here, he said, "no one sets the bar properly in terms of what is and isn't ethical."[33] He added that the most he could do was to give me "symptomatic characteristics" but that it was up to me to explore things in a systematic fashion.

Keel's company (like several others) champions risk minimization in drug development: "The recent concern over adverse events is prompting our industry to become far more vigilant in monitoring their risk-benefit profiles, before and after drug approval," he said in an emphatic way. Over time, I began to see his professional trajectory as similar to Dr. Besselaar's; both mobilized new forms of expertise at the nexus of drug development and regulation. It would have been easy to typecast Dr. Keel and his industry colleagues as mere pawns of big pharma. Engaging him and his colleagues on their own terms was a much more attractive prospect, since it permitted me to gain a better sense of the moral deliberations and actions that are possible in arenas constantly marked by the threat of negative publicity and overwhelming financial stakes.

Dr. Keel's was not a glossy pharmaceutical public relations narrative. His critiques were field-tested, sure-footed, and unconcealed. When he confronted ethical problems and scientific missteps, he reflected and acted on them and sometimes made them public. Truth speaking of this sort had a value; it shifted attention toward sponsors, and its aim was to reinvent the trial sponsor–CRO relationship. There was a place for his sort of discourse, and people in the CRO world admired him for the part he played in promoting self-regulation, skillful judgment, and advancement of his business sector. In our conversations, he pointed to multiple ordinary practices that he believed can compromise scientific integrity but that remain under the regulatory radar screen. Tem/po branded itself as opposed to these practices.

Dr. Keel said that in his experience, sponsors have acted with a "self-serving delusion." They "don't know what happens on the ground," and better-formalized communication channels were needed. Investigators also have many opportunities to exploit the enterprise. He believed that there is plenty of room to act in bad faith—increasing the costs of testing, making research less than efficient, driving it elsewhere—even if regulations are in place. A great number of patients remain relatively uninformed of these dynamics. While recent drug withdrawals have led regulators to scrutinize safety concerns more actively (Institute of Medicine 2006), Keel believed protocols remained inadequate to the task of modeling harm in the human testing phase. He went so far as to say that safety data are even destroyed:

> Take the scientific method as it applies to benefit: we have a hypothesis and then systematically structure data collected and evaluate for or against the hypothesis. But when it comes to safety, no hypotheses are articulated. They are embedded latently, but you can't recognize them in a protocol. And the data collection instrument is totally generic and not focused. It's just a matter of counting adverse effects. Whereas in benefit, it's asking a specific question in a very precise way.

The accounts that I had heard from scientists in the clinical trials industry took on a sense of urgency in 2004, when the drug rofecoxib (Vioxx) was suddenly removed from the market. Vioxx is a nonsteroidal anti-inflammatory drug (NSAID) used in treating arthritis, acute pain conditions, and dysmenorrhoea (menstrual cramping). It belongs to a class of treatments known as COX-2 selective inhibitors that target COX-2, an enzyme responsible for inflammation and pain. The withdrawal of Vioxx from the market was a major event in the pharmaceutical world. Merck, the drug's manufacturer, voluntarily withdrew it because of the drug's adverse cardiovascular effects.

COX-2 inhibitors and over-the-counter remedies such as naproxen (Aleve) work similarly in terms of relieving arthritis pain, but COX-2 inhibitors produce fewer gastrointestinal side effects (such as ulceration or bleeding). Because of this known benefit, the FDA gave Vioxx's investigational new drug (IND) application priority FDA review. Initial evaluations, however, were characterized by "the use of small, short-term trials, the exclusion of high-risk patients, and the methodologic inattention to cardiovascular events [which] minimized the possibility of uncovering evidence of cardiovascular harm" (Psaty and Furberg 2005:1134). "FDA reviewers cannot know all the facts related to a drug," I was told, "and since they can't, they will rely on precedent. They erred on the side of benefit rather than caution." An estimated 80 million people had used Vioxx since its approval in 1999; the drug's annual sales were $2.5 billion (Topol 2004:1707).

Several weeks prior to the Vioxx recall, specialists on the Data and Safety Monitoring Board, who were monitoring the safety of a clinical trial (known by the name APPROVe) meant to evaluate the efficacy of rofecoxib in the prevention of colon cancer, stopped the trial. Celecoxib (Celebrex), a competing drug in the same class of COX-2 inhibitors, had already been approved for this indication, and Merck wanted to add this to the list of indications for its product. Based on the data from the study, the monitoring board found that rofecoxib users had a higher risk of heart attacks and strokes. The safety of rofecoxib had been questioned at least since 2000, and the manufacturer, it was later revealed, had downplayed risk.[34] Critics inside and outside the agency charged that the FDA had also erred by not doing enough to assess the safety of the drug. Dr. David Graham, a director of the FDA Drug Safety Office, for example, declared "the FDA to be 'broken'" and, in his testimony in a hearing before the Senate Finance Committee, "criticized the agency for insisting on a statistically significant result before finding a safety risk" (Gilhooley 2007:953; Graham 2004). About forty-five thousand people have sued Merck, contending that they or family members have experienced heart attacks or strokes after taking Vioxx. So far, none of the plaintiffs have received payments from the company. As recently reported by the *New York Times,* "Promising to contest every case,

Merck has spent more than $1 billion over the last three years in legal fees. It has refused, at least publicly, to consider even the possibility of an overall settlement to resolve all the lawsuits at once. . . . And estimates of Merck's ultimate liability, once as high as $25 billion, are now closer to $5 billion" (Berenson 2007:A1).

For my CRO interlocutors, this and other cases served as a wake-up call to the risks and liabilities in outsourcing and of the clinical trials industry's service as foot soldiers for drug companies. As one scientific expert of a midsized CRO told me, "It used to be that, when you are a CRO, you just get handed the study protocol and do it." In this somewhat naive framing, CROs used to assume that the trial sponsor had "done its homework" in terms of ensuring the safety of volunteers in a trial, and then "you're off and running doing it." But sometimes, he added, "ethical concerns emerge only after ongoing thinking about what we are doing." Dr. Smith suggests that outsourcing contracts are incomplete in the sense that they do not fully anticipate the uncertainties that the doing of the research actually entails.

Recent drug scandals are textbook cases of how conflicts of interest can pervade the drug-testing process in both commercial and regulatory spheres. But, according to Dr. Smith, "People had seen signs of disaster, even before scandals emerged."[35] For him, they illustrate how bias is built into clinical trials to overemphasize drug efficacy and to "engineer out" evidence of potential harms, thus heightening the experimental aspect of drug use in the postapproval stage (see Gilhooley 2007:943). Such bias induction, he said with frustration, is now standard in research protocol design. Many CRO scientists I spoke with conveyed an intense commitment to the scientific method—an approach to evidence-based science that they believe is being lost as a result of the industry's "pushing toward protocol designs that maximize signs of drug benefit."

I spoke to an investigator who was part of a team conducting studies of a drug that was later taken off the market. As she recalled, "Our study was coming along. But the consulting physicians on this trial noted that overall there was a slightly higher background rate [in the combined group] of serious adverse events [SAEs]. More than one would expect. All potential cases of SAEs were documented, even if investigators thought they were not SAEs." Her team made a running list and sent the findings to the trial sponsor. "With full naïveté," the team expected the sponsor to act on the information because "it is usually scrupulous with every detail of a study." The protocol turned out to be "too dangerous to carry out on the ground." Team members recommended that the sponsor convene a scientific panel to address potential adverse effects and redesign the study to account for those effects. "We put it in writing and sent it all the way through. Once we did, we thought we had locked in the sponsor. It had to deal with the information." But the trial sponsor avoided dealing with the information and the drug was approved.

This scientist's account is one of conversion from industry steward to industry critic. And with it, she expands her company's entrepreneurial scope and scientific voice. This expert was keen to create a paper trail to note the evidence of adverse effects that her team had found. As this case reveals, outsourcing can involve implicit transfers of risk and liability that CRO subcontractors (not to mention the public) must find ways to deal with. This CRO wanted little to do with the sponsor's hazardous protocol and wanted to protect itself from regulatory action.[36] But I couldn't help thinking about what other researchers in similar positions did or did not do. From first-time investigators in the new global terrains of industry-sponsored research, I would learn that reporting an adverse event takes courage. If the adverse event is serious enough, an entire trial can be unblinded or stopped. For investigators and CROs, this might mean losing one's income or a company's contract. "We never got a contract from that manufacturer again. There is a price to be paid when you do that."

Audited records might at most reveal investigators' misconduct, but there are many more aspects to the research enterprise and its ethics that operate beyond regulatory oversight. How to address data-producing practices— packaged as ethical—that engineer out harm? The above example puts a new twist on the debate over how to best ensure safety of the country's drug supply and patient protection. Reform advocates have emphasized rooting out conflicts of interest in the FDA and making its operations more transparent, increasing postmarketing surveillance, establishing an independent drug safety agency, and creating clinical trials databases to ensure public accessibility as a means of eliminating bias in the publication of clinical trials results, which is being realized (see chapter 3). Others have called for more robust health technology assessment programs run by governments that are also primary drug purchasers (see chapter 4).

Interestingly, there has been little or no public discussion of how outsourcing and offshoring generate novel strategies of evidence making: providing new opportunities for manufacturers to create the data they want and to arbitrage it in the context of regulatory drug approval. The clinical trials industry provides a snapshot-view into the "massive arbitrage" that, according to the CEO of a leading pharmaceutical firm, "is really the definition of globalisation" (Garnier 2005:2). Disaggregating core industrial processes and rebuilding them elsewhere allows companies "to take full advantage of the massive *arbitrage . . . arbitrage* in labour cost, in financial cost, but also in pools of skilled employees and in regulatory and administrative hurdles" (ibid.). Offshored clinical development is a form of arbitrage—a hedged investment—that is meant to derive profit not only from differences in price but also from differential labor and patient costs. Arbitrage takes full advantage of imbalanced and oftentimes unjust global playing fields that are neither relative nor flat. It has become a routine tactic in organizing trials worldwide—at a time when bioethics debates about ethical practices in human subjects research and regulatory oversight mechanisms have become focused on securing procedural integrity such as informed consent.

In the words of one clinical trials expert, "There is a horrible economic disincentive to be right. So the industry is finding more Machiavellian ways to be ethical." This professional attributed the pattern of underrecognized harms in the drug supply, in part, to inadequate regulatory controls, or what he called a kind of FDA "instrumentalism." In the drug application review process, he told me, reviewers' purview is limited: "They are looking only for data on safety and efficacy, and how protocols are arranged and statistics are analyzed." One FDA reviewer likened his role to that of an air traffic controller. Air traffic controllers analyze information "that's available to them and make recommendations that can be acted on."[37] As the trials expert explained to me, "The FDA reacts upon 'evidence of,' *not the logic of how you got there.*" This instrumentalism, in the end, strengthens the hand of arbitrage and weakens the FDA's ability to assess drug efficacy and safety.

The logic of how you got there. When patient recruitment criteria are "overedited," protocol execution becomes much more complex. Study protocols can engineer up the superior effects of a study drug by increasing the adverse side effects of a competitor drug—for example, by prescribing that drug in dosages that do not reflect patterns of clinical use. Or study protocols can engineer out the potential side effects of a study drug—for example, by requiring patients on the active arms of studies to take additional therapies that will lower the chance that an adverse side effect will appear. In these instances companies do not have to provide justification; researchers carrying out a protocol are required to do it. As one researcher told me, "Firms are driven by trends in the pharmaceutical market and by the competition to prove that one medication is better than others." The "science" behind the approval of brand-name drugs can, paradoxically, make assessment of their postapproval risks more intangible. Needless to say, without such protocol tinkering, differences between newer and older drugs treating similar conditions would in many cases be narrowed substantially.

We must also place the story of the underdetection of safety problems in the wider context of tactics among companies to protect a *class* of drugs entering the market at about the same time. As anthropologist Kalman Applbaum has shown in his study of the launching of selective seratonin reuptake inhibitors (SSRIs) in Japan, companies compete against each other but they also team up to challenge and reshape health policy and medical practice, thus guaranteeing markets for an entire class of drugs. Vioxx belonged to the highly competitive class of COX-2 inhibitors. Competing companies tested similar drugs and handled the issue of cardiovascular risk differently. In one case, initial evaluation was designed to show gastrointestinal benefit as opposed to cardiovascular harm. This happened in the so-called VIGOR trial (Psaty and Furberg 2005:1133), in which rofecoxib at 50 mg once daily was compared to naproxen for up to twelve months, affording a "'worst case' estimate of the risk of serious GI bleeding for rofecoxib in comparison to naproxen" (Decision Memorandum 2005:9). The study was not designed to track possible cardiovascular hazards associated with the use of so high a dose. Other studies required patients on the active arms of trials to take low-dose aspirin: "on theoretical grounds the addition of low-dose aspirin (a COX-1 inhibitor) to a COX-2 selective drug should resolve any increased [cardiovascular] risk caused by COX-2 selectivity" (ibid.:8). But patients on low-dose aspirin *and* on the COX-2 inhibitor arm of studies lost most of the gastrointestinal benefits that COX-2 selective drugs promised. In the end, minimal reliable data are available to confirm whether COX-2 selective agents actually reduce the risk of serious gastrointestinal bleeding that is sometimes associated with older over-the-counter nonsteroidal anti-inflammatory drugs (ibid.:12).

When the realities of testing discount the realities of a tested drug's clinical use, new problems arise. The reality of direct-to-consumer marketing adds another layer of complexity to the issue of safety. As cardiologist Eric Topol writes, "Rather than a sufficient waiting period after approval to firmly establish safety in the large, representative 'real world' population, the unbridled promotion [of Vioxx] exacerbated the public health problem" (2005:367). The mismatch between the "real world" patient in a clinical setting and the highly selected, "biologically edited" patient in a clinical trial presents an ongoing challenge for evidence-based medicine.

Which brings us to offshoring. The "value" of offshoring from the perspective of trial sponsors is access to data that can facilitate drug approvals, among other things. CRO scientists are not typically in the position to pronounce judgment on the value of the drugs they test (though they have much to say about value). But they are critical of randomization strategies that focus on homogenous patient groups and that exclude real-life users. One CRO scientist offered a sobering view of globalizing trials from the perspective of safety. Noting that the "level of scientific rigor is just as good or better in other countries where our drug research takes place," the problem is the generalizability of results. "How can I generalize the data? So I've got a million patients to choose from in Eastern Europe. Now I can narrowly and homogenously define whom I use in order to pick out the right 10,000. Is that a bad thing? Is it a bad thing for the patients and the health-care community in Poland? No. But that does not mean that bad things aren't going to happen." In his view, clinical trials can create short-term benefits for local communities but long-term unknowns for end users. In the experimentality this scientist depicts, there is a conceptual blurring of the category of the human subject and consumer-citizen. Individuals are made vulnerable but in variable ways.

Distortions in the drug trial evidence base produce intangible risks and point to the relevance of contract research to public health debates over safety. Some have called for incentives for improvements in pre- and post-market testing to demonstrate initial and long-term safety and meaningful comparative advantage (Wood 2006; Gilhooley 2007). For most of the industry, preventing risk remains costly, as it would imply a reconstitution of its modus operandi (as made visible through outsourcing). Drug companies are "either setting aside money to pay out claims or developing strategies that would minimize legal and financial exposure," or they are shifting trial activities to third parties that must seriously weigh medical and legal responsibility when it comes to accepting questionable protocols. High-tech "consumer-side" solutions are also under way. But medical risks that appear to be self-generated within the current clinical trials operational model are not addressed.[38]

The Scientific Plateau and the New Safety Paradigm

The U.S. Food and Drug Administration recently developed a Critical Path Initiative with the goal of "improving the accuracy of the tests used to predict the safety and efficacy of investigational medical products."[39] While my interlocutors in the clinical trials industry agree with the basic premise of the initiative, many think that it is too focused on integrating new technologies (such as genomics and proteomics, imaging, and bioinformatics) in achieving its goals. These experts argue that the problem of safety lies in the design and conduct of clinical trials.

The federal initiative aims to reverse the "stagnation" in drug development, that is, the "recent slowdown, instead of the expected acceleration, in innovative medical therapies' reaching patients." This requires more than a high-science fix, Dr. Keel argued. The current operational model of clinical trials is incapable of scientifically predicting risk, and it needs a major overhaul. There is a "find and fix" approach by which safety and data problems are detected and fixed either during the trial or after the fact, rather than prevented beforehand. This approach consumes a lot of money, and it has not improved human subjects protection and scientific integrity: "Ten times more money is spent on 'repairing' or 'cleaning' the data than on prevention," Dr. Keel told me. Retrospective cleaning of this sort can be inherently biased, and information on safety is systematically lost.

> The industry's clinical trials process loses some 25 percent of the information content on efficacy. It loses about 90 percent of the information on harm. It's like institutional racism, a systemic bias. The industry has gone overboard consistently to figure out how to maximize signs relative to noise when it comes to showing benefit. And when it comes to harm, it is doing the bare minimum of what we need. You can look at trial after trial and see that benefit has got the most exquisite modulation you can imagine. Whereas in harm, there's no modulation.

A lot of scrutiny has been focused on study mills as the problem, said Dr. Keel, pointing with intentional irony to himself. "But the problem is more pervasive." A paradigm of expected failure informs the industry's research operations. Failure to adequately predict safety outcomes is now simply expected, he suggests. Serious adverse event reporting plans and cleaning up of "dirty data"—these are the conventional modes through which safety problems are detected in the trial phase (and they are a feature of any clinical trials agreement). But, for each protocol, pharmaceutical clients set the limits for how much verification of safety data (called source data verification) will actually take place. "At a certain point, it's all about money," I was told. An ethics focused on investigator misconduct does not necessarily capture this financial calculus over risk and safety, which seems to restrict the research process in terms of how much will be known or not known about a drug's safety profile. Given the wide latitude that pharmaceutical firms have in "governing" this evidence-making process, stagnation, in Dr. Keel's opinion, is par for the course.

The pharmaceutical industry has reached a scientific plateau. According to one clinical trials expert: "In the past thirty years, the industry has enjoyed one of the most sustained periods of scientific development. It suffered under the fantasy that it would continue like this ad infinitum—it's still under that fantasy if you read the press—but the last ten years show that it did not." This professional told me that the scientific plateau is symptomatically exposed when "a therapeutic area gets hot":

> When this happens, it's like a cattle stampede. Sponsors with different drugs compete in that therapeutic area, and this leads to a hyperdemand for investigators. And good investigators cannot compete. . . . The industry is now running out of steam. It can't get away with patent abuse through pseudo-filings in the patent law, ad infinitum price increases, me-too drugs, and product indication extensions. This is where the money and the revenue and profits from the industry were coming from. But scientific discovery has been in decline since the late eighties.

Several CRO scientists I engaged insisted that it is not enough for the industry to merely outsource drug development as a way of fighting short-term economic losses. The industry must innovate at its own peril. "So now they are squeezing down expenses. The logic is that if you squeeze CROs, and the investigators are squeezed by the CROs, and the sponsors directly squeeze the investigators, all this squeezing is going to break things down in terms of quality. We are seeing that." The intense amount of litigation the industry faces in the United States also reflects "the fundamental abandonment of the scientific method as it is not being tailored to prioritize safety. It's a lottery game."

I was told that very little money is allocated in study budgets for planning and risk prevention. To counteract the unsophisticated and haphazard sorts of error detection and repair that are in place, several CROs have taken safety as their rallying point. They advocate for a new research modus operandi that would improve productivity, lower risk, and increase scientific robustness. They want more involvement in study design, for example, and less involvement in data cleanup. Floater sites and fly-by-night experts should be purged from the research enterprise and the subjectivity of investigators reengineered. Close and comparative attention to the performance of study sites is badly needed, and high-quality data collectors should be financially rewarded.

As I showed in this chapter, CROs have increasingly differentiated themselves from the pharmaceutical industry in their scope and mission. And at this particular juncture, Dr. Keel and others are challenging the idea that they are simply doing blind recuperative work for the industry. These experts claim to be reinserting academic rigor into the drug-development enterprise. In the next two chapters, we will meet other actors who claim to be restoring scientific fidelity to clinical research. Rather than positioning themselves as isolated entrepreneurs who are being "squeezed down by costs," they reaffirm their membership in a scientific community upon which trust and integrity can be rebuilt. The industry's operational model will not change of its own volition, and the government's regulatory efforts are technocratic and remedial at best, they argue.

Dr. Keel is very selective of the trials he takes on, and his company is also taking a more active role in the design of study protocols. Risk can no longer just be deferred. Claiming safety and ethics as its territory now, the company is building up a new kind of capital, a unique selling point. The clinical trials operational model has to become—to put it simply—scientific again. But how effectively protocol redesigns and contract rearrangements can actually address potential harm, and how the "needs, interests, and rights of society" can temper a market ethics in the human subjects research enterprise, are open questions. As Hans Jonas suggests, the divorce of research from political and social realities is a constant hurdle to be overcome.

CHAPTER THREE

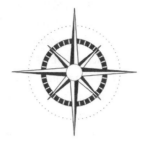

THE GLOBAL CLINICAL TRIAL

Scientists . . .
What have they left us?
Only the accountancy of a capitalist enterprise.
—*Czeslaw Milosz*[1]

How Many Clinical Trials Are Being Carried Out Worldwide?

"Unfortunately, and really quite embarrassingly, we don't know how many trials are being carried out worldwide today," Dr. Ida Sim, associate director for medical informatics at the University of California, San Francisco, told me. It was March 2006 and I was at UCSF giving a talk on offshore clinical research. Dr. Sim approached me after the talk and told me that she was co-ordinating a World Health Organization (WHO) effort to create a global databank of clinical trials (the International Clinical Trials Registry Platform, ICTRP). She and her colleagues were advocating for a comprehensive metaregister of trials and their outcomes.

This initiative was announced in November 2004, in the wake of scandals involving the suppression and selective reporting of trial results (on the antidepressant agent paroxetine, known as Paxil, for example) that benefited proprietary interests rather than serving public health risk and safety concerns (Sim and Detmer 2005:1090). Two months earlier, the International Committee of Medical Journal Editors (ICMJE) had issued a statement: "Unfortunately, selective reporting of trials does occur, and it distorts the body of evidence available for clinical decision making" (DeAngelis et al.

2004:1363). The editors declared that their journals would consider for publication only articles based on registered trials and called for the creation of an international trial registry (ibid.).[2] The WHO trial databank would be a catalyst for better evidence-based medical practice, but there would be political obstacles in the way of its creation. "We all know that on the science side, trials are gamed—not just by industry but also by academia," as one clinical trials expert had told me. Trial registration was just a first step in "shining a small light on a dark secret."

I was eager to learn about the WHO global registration effort. In my trips to Brazil, Poland, and Russia, I had learned that trial reporting practices vary greatly. The International Clinical Trials Registry Platform could provide the public with access to a field of scientific activity that is largely under the purview of industry and national regulatory bodies. Kay Dickersin, cochair of the ICTRP scientific advisory group and her colleague Drummond Rennie, deputy editor of the *Journal of the American Medical Association*, listed some of the major barriers to a comprehensive repository of clinical trials: "industry resistance, the lack of a funding appropriation for a serious and sustained effort, lack of a mechanism for enforcement of policies, and lack of awareness of the importance of the problem" (Dickersin and Rennie 2003:516).

Clinical trials offshoring is driven, in part, by cost savings and market expansion. In the process, the line between experimental and standard treatments is shifting. Concepts of vulnerability and governing rules lose force as a global data-making regime makes different groups vulnerable in different ways. We must focus on "characteristics of the research protocol and environment that present ethical challenges" (Levine et al. 2004:44). The WHO wants to see trials registered at their inception, and it wants public access to information about "ongoing, completed and published clinical trials," because such information can inform appropriate medical decision making.[3] A global databank could also help redefine research priorities, reduce duplication of research efforts, and ensure transparency in research. Likewise, a comprehensive trial register would help state and nonstate actors assess the impact that the growth of clinical research is having on national and often poor health systems. National regulatory bodies could draw from this register to better target public health needs and to improve research oversight and mechanisms of human subjects protection.

The geography of drug research and the demography of trial participants are rapidly changing, and my forays into estimates of clinical trials worldwide would find no consistency and little verifiable numerical accuracy. "Fifty thousand." One researcher working at a clinical trials intelligence firm gave me this number for the trials taking place worldwide in 2005—approximately two-thirds of them are conducted in the United States.[4] To arrive at the fifty thousand figure, this researcher and colleagues relied on FDA estimates of the number of trials initiated annually on the basis of new drug applications submitted, the number of drugs currently in development, and the average length of trials.[5] He concedes that fifty thousand is a guesstimate too— "very conservative" because the FDA data are "incomplete." Some clinical trials do not require FDA approval, such as studies of new uses of already FDA-approved drugs, provided the mechanisms of action are similar, and NSF- (National Science Foundation) and NIH-sponsored research. New drug applications that companies voluntarily withdraw are also not counted. According to the director of the largest U.S. trial databank (ClinicalTrials.gov), "only about 20% of Investigational New Drug applications result in approved drugs; this means that most trials submitted to the FDA are not eligible for inclusion" in a database of FDA-approved products (Zarin et al. 2007:2119).

I was told that when FDA drug reviewers assess an application for approval, "they typically do not know how many trials take place within a single drug application." It may be that any number of unknown trials resulted in negative or neutral findings and were tossed out. Moreover, drug reviewers can be selective in their treatment of data. "They are looking only at evidence of safety and efficacy, how the research protocols are arranged, and how the statistics are analyzed. They don't distinguish data in terms of the trial phases they are derived from, or where the data all come from. You can have one hundred Phase 2 trials for a single drug. Phase 3 trials might have various studies [with different dosages or comparison drugs] included in them."

Trials can be counted in different ways—there is no standardized format. The calculation can be based on the number of drug applications submitted to a drug regulatory agency (like the FDA), the number of trials contained in one research protocol, or the number of trials per investigational site. "If you have a multicenter trial that is conducted according to a single research protocol but in ten to twenty countries, are you counting the protocol or are you counting the number of sites involved?" As this expert suggests, estimating the number of clinical trials is an inexact science, to say the least, and those attempting to do so are faced with a complex global field of experimental activity whose true scope is largely unknown and whose operations are uncharted.

Compiling accurate estimates is complicated even further by the fact that "there are so many types of trials and so many definitions of trials." Sometimes investigators don't think of their experiments as trials, I was told. That is, distinctions between hypothesis testing and exploratory trials can blur. So, too, can distinctions between the phases of trials meant to prove drug safety and efficacy. New regulatory mechanisms make drug development shorter and more flexible. In the last two decades, for example, the FDA has launched a series of initiatives to shorten drug approval times and to hasten the public's access to experimental treatments for serious or life-threatening conditions such as HIV/AIDS. Fast-track status is highly desirable, as it allows companies to market new drugs and recoup investments before all evidentiary criteria have been met.

But these regulatory mechanisms can also compound the experimental aspects of postmarket drug use (Gilhooley 2007:954). It was believed, for example, that COX-2 inhibitors would cause fewer stomach problems than do cheaper over-the-counter pain relievers, but the priority review for Vioxx, as we now know, came at a high cost of safety. This and other instances exposed not just oversight problems in FDA review, but entrenched conflicts of interest and the urgent need to deal with regulatory loopholes and to reform drug safety standards (Institute of Medicine 2006).

The WHO database takes a radical approach to the monitoring of the global clinical trial: the goal is to register *all* studies of drugs in human beings, be they conducted on sick patients or on healthy volunteers, in *all* phases of trials. This move stands to expose the internal workings of recent drug-development strategies. For instance, to weed out poor drug candidates sooner, drug firms are making unprecedented investments in early-stage clinical testing. There has been a boom in Phase 1 (drug dosaging and safety) studies.[6] And Phase 1 trials, often doubling as proof-of-concept studies, are being retained in-house (Canavan 2008). Several experts I spoke to were alarmed by rumors about early-phase nanotechnology trials taking place in southern India, for example. "Poor people are being injected with nanytes!" We have moved a long way from the idea that a four-phase randomized control trial model could tame business interests in medicine; the principle of containment is lost in these "experiments without borders" (Jasanoff 2006).[7]

One of the largest existing clinical trials registries is the U.S. Clinical Trials.gov. In 1997, the Food and Drug Administration Modernization Act (FDAMA), section 113, mandated the registration of all new drug efficacy trials for "serious and life-threatening diseases," and this mandate led to the creation of ClinicalTrials.gov.[8] The databank, which is maintained by the

National Institutes of Health, was first made publicly available via the Internet in early 2000; it offers updated information on enrollment in federally and privately supported clinical research. Its scope has widened to include other types of trials, and today it contains listings from all over the world. In an essay on the need for a global trial databank, Sim and Detmer took note of the critical fact that while registration was mandatory, "only 48 percent of industry-sponsored trials were registered during the initial period of the law's implementation" (2005:1090). Moreover, trials are often registered with uninformative data, thus compromising transparency. Among industry-sponsored studies, "[e]ven when local laws require that trials be registered, compliance has been incomplete" (ibid.).

In November 2005, ClinicalTrials.gov listed 22,641 clinical studies sponsored by industry and federal agencies. Industry-sponsored trials constituted only one-quarter of the trials listed. A year later, the number of trials had increased by more than 10,000. Again, of all trials registered, only one-quarter were industry sponsored. This is a curious recurrence, given the fact that more than half of all clinical research projects are industry sponsored—the taxpayer-funded NIH pays for 28 percent, and private groups and universities cover the rest. The one-quarter pattern suggests significant underregistration. Moreover, when I checked both in 2005 and in 2006, ClinicalTrials.gov indicated that more than half of its listed trials took place in the United States. This pattern, again, does not correspond to the present operations of the industry. For example, a third of GlaxoSmithKline's trials currently take place in low-income countries. The company's CEO declared that offshoring would increase by 50 percent in 2007 (Cherry 2005:66).

Industry-organized trial registries have grown, but they are inconsistently organized and use "sponsor-specific proprietary software," preventing the emergence of a coherent picture (Lemmens and Bouchard 2007: 40). Yet a comprehensive metaregister of all trials—institutional resistances notwithstanding—is now feasible from a bioinformatics standpoint, and registration appears to be taking off (Laine et al. 2007). The International Clinical Trials Registry Platform encourages principal investigators or sponsors of trials to register their studies in a regional, national, or international register that would forward this data directly to the WHO. By collecting and analyzing data from twenty registration criteria, the WHO's registry would provide a public record of the health problems being studied and the countries where research is under way, the identity of the intervention (and placebo and comparator controls being used), key subject inclusion and exclusion criteria, target sample size (the number of subjects the study plans to enroll), and anticipated primary and secondary outcomes (trial results). But the industry has objected to some of the registration criteria, arguing that in order to maintain competitive advantage, firms must retain the right to withhold, at least for some time, the name of the intervention, as well as anticipated outcomes and target sample sizes. Reveal the target sample size in a given location, the industry argues, and you give competitors the chance to identify proprietary facets of protocol design and the statistical powers needed to achieve a desired outcome.[9] On the other hand, human testing is the most expensive portion of drug development. Knowing target sample sizes or how many subjects are involved in trials used to approve new drugs is crucial to accurately assessing the overall cost of developing a new drug (Light 2008:325).[10]

Much, obviously, is at stake. During an open commentary period (prior to a formal meeting among all stakeholders in the platform, held in Geneva in April 2006), industry representatives wrote letters protesting the registration of *all* trials, including, especially, early-phase trials. Raising the specter of a threat to public safety, they argued that disclosure of early-phase trials would create dangerous confusion—desperate patients might equate early-phase trial results with actual treatment. Thus required registration of trials would "hurt" public health. As the debates wore on, and as the industry began to sense its position weakening, it ratcheted up the argument against disclosure, claiming that this requirement would undercut "the sovereignty of world-wide regulatory authorities empowered to make value-based decisions for their citizens."[11] The drug company representatives not only complained of potential intellectual property theft; they branded the WHO initiative as out of legal bounds: "[W]e must be assured that external entities, working out-side the law, do not act to disrupt the economic basis of our industry."[12] Skeptics of this position note that companies "generally know what their rivals are working on," thus "competitive advantage would not be seriously affected if all companies were obliged to register all trials" (Godlee 2006:1108).

The industry's reaction to the open-source initiative is not surprising. Perhaps more striking is the reluctance of major regulatory bodies to engage the effort. When a company registers a trial on ClinicalTrials.gov, it submits a code number that conceals the product's identity but that should corre-spond to the code number as it appears on an investigational new drug (IND) application. The WHO team is coordinating its activities with Clinical Trials.gov, whose registry staff is attempting to verify protocol data that drug firms provide to ClinicalTrials.gov and to determine whether those data match with the data they supply to the FDA. Deborah Zarin, the director of the ClinicalTrials.gov team, and colleagues note that the FDA "uses its own internal identification system that is never made publicly available" (2007:2116). The agency has been slow to assist in this verification effort, as proprietary issues have not been resolved. "[W]ithout access to trial protocols it is not possible to determine, with complete certainty, that all data are accurate" (2115). Zarin et al. write, "Without the ability to validate entries, selective reporting of trial results could still occur" (2118). Companies registering new investigational products on ClinicalTrials.gov have also been known to change their serial numbers or use various serial numbers, names, or aliases (2116)—this gives them the opportunity to select which trials to publish. The inability to properly identify agents also raises safety concerns: "Serial numbers (and trials) of drugs that are never approved may remain 'masked' in the database" (2117). This means that persons searching ClinicalTrials.gov cannot access relevant safety information in prior research or its possible links to other investigative agents being studied (ibid.).

The International Clinical Trials Registry Platform is not an endpoint but a means of minimizing bias in clinical medicine and providing information upon which consumers, physicians, and regulators alike can make "value-based" treatment decisions. It aims to restore public trust in the research enterprise. And if successful, this bioinformatics venture could help to crystallize a scientific culture founded on sound evidence-based medicine and the idea of a "universally valid knowledge as a public good."[13] The database is just the beginning. There will be more oversight coming down the pike. "The journals want whole protocols reported, and I think that trial registration is moving toward requiring that whole protocols and their amendments be declared. Then, the rest of us can really go in and critique everything that's been published," a reform-minded scientist told me.

In sum, the registration of all trials would enable multiple parties to assess the value of research pursuits in different contexts, and this comparative endeavor would benefit study participants, patients, global populations, and the clinical research process.[14] Along these lines, Fiona Godlee, editor of the *British Medical Journal*, writes: "To make informed decisions, participants in trials need to understand the whole landscape of other ongoing trials, not just those known to one company. Patients need to be aware of ongoing trials internationally when deciding about treatments, especially those who have run out of current treatment options. Ethics committees and institutional review boards need to know what other trials are ongoing when deciding whether to approve a new trial. Access to information is especially important for people in the developing world, where the potential for exploitation is greatest" (2006:1108).

Clinical trials also serve as a form of marketing. Long after sponsors have calculated that a drug works for a particular indication (or reason to prescribe), they continue to recruit subjects and investigators into trials as a way of promoting their product and building brand loyalty (see chapter 4). Redundancies and inefficiencies of this sort are a "necessary" part of competitive business models, but perhaps at the expense of better ones. We do not know the number of subjects involved in marketing trials, in part because we do not know how specific companies distinguish between R&D expense and marketing expense (Light 2008:325). In addition to accounting for instances of exploitation and risk in individual patient-consumers, advocates see the WHO platform as an instrument for creating a more balanced global health research agenda that addresses the needs of industrialized countries and the disease burden of the majority poor.

As clinical trials insinuate themselves into the slipstream of the global economy, trial sponsors find windows of opportunity but remain unaccountable to the complex local realities they help to engender. Doctors and patients are left to navigate these realities once the ethics question has been "papered over" (Jacob and Riles 2007). Driven by pharmaceutical capital, they depend upon public health institutions and occasion a mix of short-term care, hope, and profit. They last for some time, until regulatory regimes mature, become "excessively formal," and/or tax costs of trials increase and "pose barriers to industry development."[15] Trial entrepreneurs see the clinical research environments they help to construct as having distinct phases of evolution (opportunism, peak, "saturation," and exhaustion). Experimental landscapes then disappear and reemerge elsewhere, in another country struggling to find its place in the global economy. This hypermobility pressures national regulators who must somehow balance the needs and demands of industry, so as to make their country investor friendly, and the needs and demands of their medically underserved constituents. This chapter explores an expanding research enterprise and how it moves in a way that no trial registry, not even a global one, would necessarily capture. The clinical trials industry is highly regulated, and the quality of its performance is defined by regulation. Yet the new international and national sites in which this industry functions are not neatly layered socio-legal fields but are, rather, "distinct and even disconnected legal and political topograph[ies]" (Greenhouse 2006:190). How to reconcile images of hypermobility with the kinds of barriers to growth and liabilities encountered on the ground?

I had talked to several professionals of a contract research organization that I shall refer to as AR/CH. The firm had dozens of worldwide affiliates, including a thriving one in Poland. This affiliate office covered operations for Central and Eastern Europe and Eurasia. According to one of the company's executives, Poland was their best investment yet. The country offered highly trained professionals who "produced high-quality data and aggressively engaged the research enterprise." And this was "consistent with their capitalistic ethos." Poland "grabbed clinical research with a vengeance."

After having reached its peak in the global trial market, the country was now at a crossroads, facing new regulations that came with European Union (EU) membership. In observing transitions to an EU-harmonized operational environment, I could track how clinical trials markets rise and fall, and what comes after them. I interviewed many professionals (executives, trial managers, physicians, lawyers, and policy makers) who had made Poland an extremely efficient clinical trials destination and others who were engaged in similar work in nearby countries. In speaking with these professionals, I inquired into larger questions: Which economic strategies underlie this offshored trial movement? What kinds of infrastructures and collaborations help to foster clinical research environments? What public functions, other than evidence gathering, do clinical trials assume? How do regulations operate locally to protect patients, and which practices escape these regulations?

My inquiry into offshored trials echoes sociologist Bruno Latour's call for "making things public" (2005). In an era of global markets, technology, ecological crises, and terrorism, people are interconnected to be sure, but they aren't necessarily brought together by any shared politics or civics. We need to reimagine political assembly out of the diverse assemblages of which we are now a part: to make politics with the right objects. According to Latour, political philosophy has traditionally delineated the procedures that keep political orders—be they republics or national and international orders—intact. But the field has "been the victim of a strong object-avoidance tendency": "From Hobbes to Rawls, from Rousseau to Habermas, many procedures have been devised to assemble the relevant parties, to authorize them to contract, to check their degree of representativity, to discover the ideal speech conditions, to detect legitimate closure, to write the good constitution. But when it comes down to *what* is at is-sue, namely the object of concern that brings them together, not a word is uttered ... [T]heir *res publica* does not seem to be loaded with too many *things*" (2005:15–16).

This strong object-avoidance tendency rings powerfully true when reflecting on how little knowledge of the global clinical trial is made public—and on how essential an international trial registry is in addressing this deficit. We know very little about how experimental sites and trials are organized as economic activities, the contingent ways these sites and trials operate, and how clinical research becomes a public matter (or not). Poland, an initial key country for offshored clinical trials, is a good place to examine factors that restrict or promote the movement of the research enterprise, the bureaucratic actions that can slow down or speed up research, and the ways in which systems of human protection are imagined on the ground. Ethnography serves as one further check against the bureaucratic and technical circuitry that assists global experimentality; it also marks the place where public policy has failed to account for the liabilities and risks that are entailed in this enterprise.

The Polish Market and the "Nonexistent" Patient

For the clinical trials industry, Poland was a highly desirable country, a gateway to other research frontiers in Central-Eastern Europe and Eurasia. The technical and professional excellence of its investigators and clinical sites were well-known and prized. Patient recruitment was recognized as well structured and integrated with public health institutions. The country's central registry of clinical trials shows that from 1994 to 2000, the number of new trials registered annually grew from about seventy-five to more than four hundred. In 2003, Poland had one of the world's highest numbers of investigators active in FDA-regulated research. A major auditing firm estimated that drug companies invest roughly $322 million in clinical research in Poland each year, suggesting that clinical trials have become an important source of the country's health-care delivery.[16]

After working with independent clinical research associates for several years, AR/CH upgraded its operations in Poland. With about thirty staff members, the CRO was small compared with major competing companies. The competition for Polish sites was fierce. Still, AR/CH judged the Polish investment a worthwhile risk. A medical director of a multinational drug company that contracts with AR/CH told me that Central-Eastern Europe was "after the United States, the second largest producer of clinical data" for his company.

Poland's move from a centrally planned to a free-market economy and, recently, to EU membership has been largely hailed as a hard-won success. With its democratic turn in 1989, the country adopted a painful "shock therapy" approach—the state withdrew price controls, regulations, and subsidies to state-owned industries, and liberalized trade.[17] Inflation rose to 500 percent by 1990. The International Monetary Fund and the World Bank intervened, offering stabilization funds and credits for modernizing Polish goods and exports. While unemployment remained high, by 1992 inflation had decreased to 43 percent; and by the end of 2001 it had fallen below 4 percent. In the meantime, the private business sector flourished. Six hundred thousand new private firms were created, employing some 1.5 million people. But success is a relative term. With a population of 40 million, Poland's unemployment level remains the highest in the European Union, though its annual growth rate has been one of the highest of all former communist economies.[18] Legal and bureaucratic obstacles as well as corruption are seen as hampering this sector's further development.

Under communism, Poland was a major producer of pharmaceuticals for Eastern European states, and in the early nineties this exporting continued. By the mid-1990s, with a change in taxation policies, the country saw a major inflow of Western drugs. The Polish state pharmaceutical firm Polfa was privatized, and soon drug exports to eastern neighbors collapsed. Today, more than 60 percent of Poland's pharmaceutical market is controlled by foreign companies. Imports undercut the competitive and price-lowering prospects of their Polish equivalents.[19]

According to AR/CH scientists, the quality level of data coming from Polish research sites was exceptional; this quality allowed for efficient drug application filing. In one conversation in October 2004, I told an AR/CH executive whom I shall call Dr. Jane Francis that I would be very interested in learning about how the efficiency and excellence she spoke of were shaped on the ground. How did the global research enterprise insert itself into Poland's state and market reforms and ongoing debates over the role of public institutions? How does this capitalist enterprise account for itself? What else besides the accountancy do trials leave behind in a new Poland? I also wanted this inquiry to be of value to advocates of a transparent global trial registry.

Dr. Francis was quite concerned with the sustainability of the Polish success story, particularly with the out-migration of talent to Western Europe.

She agreed to facilitate my entry into Poland's clinical trials world and promptly telephoned a Polish associate. She connected me with a former physician whom I will call Dr. Jan Mazur, who was overseeing AR/CH's eastward expansion. In our teleconference, Dr. Mazur came across as amiable and eager to share his experiences. He and Dr. Francis worked closely together, and he had no qualms about tempering her enthusiasm for the region. He was realistic and cautious, pointing to weaknesses in the system that his expertise could and could not remediate. In fact, by 2006, the Polish clinical trials market went on the decline. Among industry observers, it had gotten a reputation of posing excessive regulatory and tax barriers: "Since joining the European Union the conditions for conducting clinical trials . . . in Poland have deteriorated significantly."[20] Dr. Mazur would be my compass, guiding me through the particularities of these conditions; he offered a firsthand look at the challenges clinical trials scientists faced in maintaining their market.

Dr. Mazur had completed his medical training at one of Poland's most prestigious medical schools and worked at its hospital as a cardiologist. He was also employed in the public health sector and worked with elderly populations. In the mid-1990s, he left medical practice and became an independent clinical research associate for a European-based entrepreneur who procured trial sites and patients in Central-Eastern Europe. As one of Poland's first native trial monitors, he worked as a freelancer for AR/CH and trained a new cohort of experts. His successes led to offers of more lucrative positions within the U.S. offices of the company, but, as he told me in June 2005 when I visited Warsaw, he preferred the pleasures of his hometown and the cosmopolitanism of traveling in Europe and Asia.

In her book *Privatizing Poland*, anthropologist Elizabeth Dunn explores how Polish food production became linked to global markets in the transition from socialism to neoliberal capitalism. New management techniques such as accounting, audit, and quality control standards constituted the "quiet backbone" of the transition project, and new ideas of personhood were instantiated. Flexible and self-regulating workers were needed to help firms to compete in global markets yet, in practice, these disciplinary techniques hybridized with social relationships that marked everyday survival under socialism (Dunn 2004:7). One could describe Dr. Mazur as both a representative and a vector of such transformations in the trial industry's labor force. He trained scores of clinical research associates and new investigators and instituted rigid job-performance evaluations.

Dr. Mazur introduced me to his long-standing collaborators, grouping them into those he said he "trusted" and those who "required too much monitoring." He spoke of "overeager" investigators who wanted to use the system for "immediate benefit" or who relaxed eligibility requirements to enroll more patients, and thus jeopardized the outcome and sustainability of the enterprise. Some investigators were too sympathetic toward their patients and had a tendency to overenroll them for medical care purposes. These persons—potential "protocol-violators"—had to be weeded out. As Dr. Mazur spoke, I was reminded of Dunn's observation that some Poles were too embedded in social relations and incapable of self-management: "new kinds of persons and subjectivities had to be created" (2004:6). His was a technical mission. Human relations and the moral and cultural environment had to be tamed, traditional doctor-patient relations remolded, so that reliable data could be guaranteed. Dr. Mazur told me,

> Our mission is not about treating the patient. This is not a primary objective, and somehow this is explicitly forbidden. Investigators can recruit only eligible patients. It's the physician's decision as to who will be participating. But maybe this patient has a more severe disease; that's a secondary consideration. Patients must meet the inclusion/exclusion criteria first. Other factors are informal, whether he wants to help this or that patient. But this decision has to be guided by the protocol. *We don't see patients, we see data.*

I asked Dr. Mazur what had brought him to his work. There were two turning points in his life and medical career in the mid-1990s. First, his brother was diagnosed with a fatal blood disorder, and Dr. Mazur enrolled him in a clinical trial. Though his sibling passed away shortly thereafter, he told me that this experience led him to see the therapeutic value of trials. As a cardiologist, Dr. Mazur was well connected to the best specialists in public hospitals. Thus he was able to offer his brother what he considered state-of-the-art medicine, still a scarce commodity in an overburdened and somewhat isolated health-care system. This experience made him rethink the very idea of patienthood. In the socialist system, he told me, a patient was a "passive recipient" of health. In a capitalist system, a patient was an agent of his or her own care: "At least you now have the chance to improve, provided you take responsibility." The idea of the socialist patient as passive is not entirely consistent with the facts. Poles, like other socialist citizens, engaged in informal practices of exchanges and favors in the context of chronic shortage. These systems of exchange continue and can exclude many from timely public health access.[21] Trial access offers an alternative to this system. Alluding to professional networks and using a discourse of self-reliance, agency, and responsibility, Dr. Mazur translated his family tragedy into the morality that underpins his work.

The second turning point also came at the time of his brother's illness, when Dr. Mazur began making his first forays into subject recruitment, working as a freelance recruiter for two small European companies. As his clinical research network expanded, he became known for his reliability and efficiency. He then left medical practice and dedicated himself, with self-assertiveness and pride, to working full-time as one of Poland's first clinical research associates. He was confident in his quality-assurance role. He had everything to be proud of and nothing to hide.

In 2003, AR/CH promoted Dr. Mazur to director of regional development. As new protocols arrive on Dr. Francis's desk in the United States, she asks Dr. Mazur to help her assess the feasibility of launching the trials in Poland. In Dr. Mazur's words, "Jane has a wide view of the feasibility and performance of sites. She knows that a small percentage of the sites will recruit the majority of the patients globally, so she is very systematic in trial placement."

Dr. Mazur is very good at marketing his country and region. He produces informational Webcasts to potential clients and AR/CH's marketing team. I first met Dr. Mazur in person in early 2004, when he visited the company's headquarters to discuss ongoing and future projects. We reviewed plans for my summer trip to Warsaw, and he invited me to attend a presentation he was to give that day. In the presentation, he covered epidemiological and economic data as well as information on the Polish health-care system and clinical trials market. The message was clear: here you will not fail in recruiting, and you will get reliable data. To my dismay, under the slide "fast recruitment," he showed an image of long lines of people queued up for consumer items. As if they were still living in a socialist-type shortage economy, I thought, and as if trials were a way of circumventing shortages in the present. The image emphasized the extent to which the industry brings together very unequally positioned actors—patients whose medical options are limited and physicians whose economic possibilities are open.

Poised and self-assured, Dr. Mazur portrayed the Polish health-care system as in disarray and clinical trials as only doing good. Among the points he mentioned were these: the infant death rate is higher in Eastern Europe than the EU average, and overall life expectancy is lower. In Poland there are many advanced-stage cancer and diabetes patients, both previously untreated and with limited access to specialized treatments. Cardiovascular and respiratory diseases are highly prevalent, and the costs of chronic-disease treatments are a huge burden on diminishing public health budgets.

Poland's universal health-care system remains poorly financed; employees make large contributions to the state health insurer. Seventy percent of the cost of drugs is paid out of pocket—the highest percentage in the European Union. Hospital costs are not reimbursed, and the level of preventive medicine is generally low. Dr. Mazur juxtaposed these dire data with information about the high quality of the clinical research environment and its adaptation to international standards. Global FDA inspections data corroborate this assessment of high quality, he argued. Even though Central-Eastern European sites have been the object of much less FDA scrutiny than their North American and Western European counterparts, they have yielded the lowest "finding per FDA inspection ratio." Central-Eastern European sites compete with Latin American sites. The latter, Dr. Mazur noted, have the highest "finding per FDA inspection ratio"—that is, more protocol violations, falsification of data, and informed consent noncompliance, and poor adverse event reporting.

The clinical trials enterprise relies on the work of professionals such as Dr. Mazur who navigate both the public and private health-care sectors. As in most transitioning economies, many doctors in Poland work in public health but also have private practices, and a growing number have migrated into other types of medical-industry work. Dr. Mazur assured the audience at AR/CH that Poland had a highly skilled clinical research labor force. In recent years, the Polish staff of monitors has grown by 30–40 percent annually, and more than half of AR/CH's personnel in the region have medical degrees. And although Polish patients are, as Dr. Francis told me, "beginning to cost the same as Western European patients," AR/CH has concluded that the benefits of clinical research—in terms of guaranteed recruitment and excellence of data—still outweigh the cost.

Dr. Mazur related success stories in his presentation. One such story involved a placebo-controlled study for a diabetes drug. The study's inclusion criteria required previously untreated patients with "very high" blood-sugar levels. One of his PowerPoint slides read, "This is a difficult medical condition. This high-risk patient population is almost nonexistent." The focus of the study was a me-too drug. With minimal pharmacological alteration, me-too drugs exploit well-established markets. Their trials require large numbers of patients and by and large produce little or no evidence of additional therapeutic gain. Given the severity of the condition and the strictness of the study's subject-inclusion criteria, not surprisingly initial recruitment was low, said Dr. Mazur. The manufacturer hired AR/CH to "rescue" the trial. Dr. Mazur was called in, and the study was redesigned. Inclusion criteria were relaxed to include patients with a slightly less severe condition. Dr. Mazur explained that "because of the complexity of this protocol," AR/CH made an unprecedented decision to hire its own physicians to review every patient already randomized to make sure each could actually receive the study treatment (or the placebo). In the end, the new Central-Eastern European sites recruited more than half of the required patients. From then on, the pharmaceutical sponsor "placed the majority of sites in our region," concluded Dr. Mazur.

When I got to Poland six months later, however, Dr. Mazur expressed concern about this success story, that is, about pressures to recruit what he referred to as "dangerously sick patients." This time he added the qualifier "dangerous" in reference to the patients whom he had previously characterized as a "high-risk population." In the global clinical trial, someone has to turn danger into an acceptable high risk. Dr. Mazur seemed reluctant to exercise this kind of expertise. Because the diabetic compound under study was a me-too drug, the protocol's aim was narrow—"to catch minor differences," he said. Having a very selective high-risk patient group would allow the number of variables affecting trial results to be minimized and would guarantee the "success" of the trial. Crucially, the patients were both dangerously ill and unexposed to other medicines for diabetes. This meant that the biochemical actions of competitor drugs would not interfere in the results and thus could be completely excluded.

"Complicated protocols are on the rise," stressed Dr. Mazur. The pursuit of insignificant and minute differences leads to the recruitment of "very, very selected patient populations." Even though he facilitated such trials, he said they were "highly unrealistic" in their demands: "Sometimes sponsors want patients that don't even exist!" He had to make such subjects come into existence, and this was indeed a high-risk venture for him and for his team. "It is dangerous, if you provide an experimental treatment to someone who should not get it or who should be getting something else."

High blood-sugar levels are accompanied by "very severe and dangerous symptoms," he added. "It becomes very difficult to exclude other causes for the same symptoms." The margin of possible error was great, and he was very concerned with controlling the experiment on the ground. Within the parameters of his work, Dr. Mazur was extremely conscientious, and his company valued him for it. Yet I could not help but wonder what others in the same position may or may not choose to do, and what harms might accrue to patients. Dangerously compromised patients remain at the mercy of a self-regulating clinical trials market. Dr. Mazur's story suggested that there is too much latitude here for variability. Recruiting physicians have room to maneuver, and therein lies the potential for risky practices that, as Dr. Mazur pointed out, can include the use of "highly edited" patients and/or treating a population that should already have been treated.

Liability issues compound Dr. Mazur's distress. The company is ostensibly safe from liability concerns if the local institutional review board approves the protocol and patients sign the informed consent forms. But Dr. Mazur has to train his study monitors to be doubly vigilant of the local Polish investigators they oversee. If an "overeager" investigator recruits the wrong patient, he "breaks" with the protocol, and either he or the CRO that hired him may be liable for injury (the division of liability is assessed case by case). The drug manufacturer has the upper hand. In addition to not being liable, it can float its protocol elsewhere—to another CRO, to another country, to another IRB—if AR/CH decides to reject it. Professionals like Dr. Mazur attenuated the dangers of protocols—making them doable without jeopardizing their region's privileged position in the clinical trials market.

"Can you filter out these dangerous protocols?" I asked.

For him and his company, the only way of reducing "exposure to danger" was to institute more selective criteria and more rigorous technical analysis of protocols: "Our company has a medical review team in our U.S. headquarters. The sponsor makes requests for a protocol bid. The protocol is carefully reviewed and we discuss it, whether it is feasible or not, whether it is better to drop it, whether it is unethical at first glance." In the meantime, on the ground, Dr. Mazur said, there was ever more vigilance and "effort to make it right": "You have to monitor very carefully whether the patients included in the study are *actually eligible*. The wrong people may get into the trial. It's a safety issue." He was convinced that all these efforts to make protocols safe were driving up the cost of drugs: "More time, more complexity, and higher prices for medications." In the end, striving for a safer experiment temporarily calms the waters and keeps such volatile and ethically sealed endeavors in the country, but at any given moment, study protocols and trials might move elsewhere.

Clinical Research Frontiers

AR/CH relies on a Southeast European subcontractor, a small firm that I will call Scop|e, to run trials there. Scop|e advertises itself as knowing local customs and having connections to drug regulatory agencies. It was founded in 2002 by an American businessman whom I refer to as Curt Johns, and who served as the marketing and sales director for a Croatian-based pharmaceutical firm. Dr. Mazur had begun to work closely with Johns and was enthusiastic about his new partner: "He has a real American work ethic."

Johns claims to have recruited more than three hundred investigators in his region. In 2005, he told me that his business was doing well. "The region had been underexplored." His company benefited from the fact that the industry "likes to distribute its large trials across different countries." Johns's trial sites have never been FDA audited, he told me. Part of his job, he suggested, was to expand trials beyond more standardized, regulated, and costly environments (EU-harmonized Poland, for example).

Frontiers are not merely a matter of geography. They are also flexible environments, where regulations are still configuring and resources (read: accessible patients) are freed up (Tsing 2004:30).[22] The Balkan countries, for example, are not subject to the European Union Clinical Trial Directive, which introduced stringent regulatory requirements for all phases of study in human subjects. This will undoubtedly change with EU expansion. Scop|e states plainly the advantages of launching trials in the Balkans *now* as it removes logistical and legal obstacles: trial sponsors do not have to be legally registered in Southeastern Europe to start up research, and Scop|e requires only a letter of designation in which sponsors delegate all trial-related duties and responsibilities to the company to which the trial is outsourced.[23]

In some ways, these new trial countries are valued as part of a "bygone" regulatory time—not yet fully matured in terms of the requirements of a harmonized technological zone (Barry 2001), but on the way. Unlike the situation an EU-regulated environment, pharmaceutical and biotechnology companies can transfer responsibility for obligations linked to a trial (including the cost of compliance with specific regulations) to EU-compliant CROs. Smaller firms like Scop|e gain footholds in the trial market by promising cost-pressured CROs that they will assume trial-related duties. They maximize efficiency and minimize the risk of their operations through their knowledge of local customs and connections to drug regulatory agencies. In this frontier, responsibility for the conduct of the trial and for insurance, along with civil liability, is continuously transferred to third parties who would in practice prove difficult to track. From the perspective of intermediary CROs, this chain of transfer is not as flexible as it may seem. Since CROs bear the cost of regulatory compliance, they have the most to lose if compliance falls short (particularly among new investigators). They have to find ways to overcome the uncertainties, financial and legal, that come with their own subcontracting.

When I asked one former regulatory officer about how to best globalize research oversight, his response conveyed that he was unaware of the realities described above. In speaking of trial expansion to the middle- and low-income countries, he said, "People there know what's right and wrong. They'll make the same mistakes we did in the United States and learn from them, just as we did." A kind of developmental arc of ethical thinking was presupposed, and investigators new to the trial enterprise were assumed to sit on its lower, less developed, end.

Dr. Francis, who plays a key role in decisions regarding AR/CH's expansion, spoke to me candidly about the company's efforts to manage the risks of their own growth. She considered her company's efforts to be far superior to the pharmaceutical industry's practice of "dumping trials," enabling them to proceed without adequate oversight. "No doubt," she said, "there is a problem with corporate governance on a global scale. If we are not sure whether a trial can be operationalized, we tend to use the support of local subcontractors. But we provide project control and oversight and would never subcontract without central oversight."

AR/CH is making the provision of oversight a central business focus in new regions. More than 60 percent of the money trial sponsors pay to CROs in Eastern Europe is related to clinical research monitoring—that is, to paying someone like Dr. Mazur and his staff to oversee the day-to-day operations of clinical trials. Even in frontier zones, trials must follow the provisions of the International Conference on Harmonisation of Technical Requirements for Registration of Pharmaceuticals for Human Use (ICH) and the Good Clinical Practice (GCP) guidelines. Launched in 1990 by regulators and research-based industry, the ICH has established uniform technical requirements and standards (such as randomized controlled trials) for international drug testing and registration. The GCP is a set of World Health

Organization guidelines for the design, conduct, performance, monitoring, auditing, recording, analysis, and reporting of clinical trials. First published in 1995, the GCP is now the industry standard, providing "assurance that the data and reported results are credible and accurate, and that the rights, integrity, and confidentiality of trial subjects are protected."[24] The timing of the legalization of the ICH-GCP guidelines varied across countries. Beginning in 1997, when a national law on medical experimentation took effect in Poland, local CROs could use their legally sanctioned position to subcontract trials to neighboring countries where ICH-GCP guidelines were not yet in place. Though drawn from less regulated environments, data collection can be mediated by a CRO stationed in an ICH-GCP country.

The ICH-GCP provides a unified standard for the European Union countries, Japan, and the United States and makes data from new research sites transferable to regulatory bodies in these major pharmaceutical markets. As a transparent and investor-friendly legal mechanism, it gives countries outside these markets the chance to participate in the clinical trials industry, and it permits the participation of even more peripheral countries as well. The large investments in clinical trials monitoring are what make this industry expansion possible. In fact, the GCP spawned a new subindustry of trial monitors, who are hired by sponsors or CROs to check documentation to make sure studies are conducted according to the protocol.

As sociologist Andrew Barry writes, harmonization of standards "depends not just on written statements and procedures, but also on the transfer and monitoring of practical skills. Harmonization is apparently a rationalistic and legalistic enterprise; but to be successful it demands the presence of persons" (2001:78). In my foray into the Eastern European trial landscape, one professional directed me to another, and so on and so on. Each person, confident in his/her specific expertise, emphasized the efficacy, seamlessness, and transparency of the whole enterprise. Trial monitors constitute the bulk of AR/CH's staff in Eastern Europe. These monitors are critical to ensuring the inflow of finance capital and the outflow of products (data) from new or untested research areas. Taken together, the practices of the skilled, the efficient, and the well-paid (many of them vocal as to the dilemmas they face) make for a less risky investment environment. These experts ensure proper documentation of informed consent and trial procedures and create an audit trail. In frontier zones, their enterprise compensates for weak or withdrawn political and legal institutions. In the end, their work is not just about capturing bodies for research but also about maintaining the value of the evidence being produced. "CROs exist because sponsors need them" (ClinPage 2007). They flourish, in part, because their monitoring protects the value of data. In doing so, however, they navigate an awkward world filled with risky actors (overeager investigators or dubious subcontractors). As they tread across steep grades of inequality, a field of experimental activity takes form—sometimes beyond what regulations can control and even account for.

A medical director of a multinational drug firm operating in Eastern Europe conceded that working with CROs is quite expensive, and that the benefits "are uneven," but asserted that "the monitoring here is better than in Western Europe. It is better because it is excessive. We can afford this excess because costs are still lower here." This surfeit of monitoring adds credibility to the data that are sent to corporate headquarters. Frontier zones and their monitoring have a special place in the contemporary economics of evidence making—and, as I was told, "the benefit of excessiveness outweighs the cost." But this model of cost-effectiveness of data gathering promulgates a very narrow conception of patient rights and corporate social responsibility. It eclipses the issue of the medical inequality that leads people to use trials as a health-care surrogate in the first place, while the quality of public health-care erodes. This professional considered himself and his company to be acting socially responsibly in this void. "We provide drugs after most projects if they are not available locally [in open label extension studies] for those who wish to participate in them. There is also compassionate use." But this type of assistance is sporadic. "We decide with investigators on a case-by-case basis. There are no rules here."[25]

Collaborations in Global Science

On a Sunday afternoon in early June 2005, I arrived in Warsaw, a city striving to shed the architecture of its socialist past: it boasts a new modern airport, glistening high-rise hotels and corporate office buildings, billboards, and congested street traffic. Warsaw and its inhabitants were all but annihilated in World War II.[26] Many of the bombed-out buildings, particularly in its Old City, were completely rebuilt. Postwar city planners were determined to faithfully replicate the destroyed originals, without a hint of romanticism about ruins or any sense of the victimization they can convey. The use of new, prefabricated materials gave the Old City's baroque homes, medieval castle, old town market square, and cathedral a curious, denatured, and almost cardboard-like presence.

I rented an apartment in a semiremodeled area in Warsaw's center, not far from Marszalkowska Street (Ulica Marszałkowska), the site of a gay pride parade scheduled for later in the month. The parade ultimately was banned by Warsaw's conservative mayor at that time, Lech Kaczyński.[27] According to some of my acquaintances there, Poland's political parties are a mix of free-marketers, economic nationalists, Europhobes, and Europhiles. Many blame the country's neoliberal policies and nonregulated markets for having delivered lowered living standards, high unemployment, and political and economic insecurity.[28] The country was dominated by a populist right-wing party that was liberal on economic issues but conservative on social ones. In my strolls through parks and malls and in conversations with locals, I perceived a deep struggle over political belonging amid religious fervor, demand for rights, and the obstacles in the way of social mobility. Poles radiated a generalized discontent with what they sensed as their lower status in the EU and major disputes over how to account for the carnage of World War II in Poland.

A few days into my stay, I met Dr. Mazur for lunch at a Thai restaurant near his office. He was eager to help, quickly jotting down the names of persons for me to contact. All of them—former public health leaders, pharmaceutical sector workers, medical directors of multinational companies, contracted physician-investigators, and drug-industry-sponsored lawyers engaged in clinical trials contract negotiation—would give me a window into the industrial research complex in the region. Dr. Mazur referred to many of his colleagues as "pioneers." According to the *Oxford English Dictionary*, the French word *pion(n)ier* denotes a foot soldier, or "one of a body of foot-soldiers who march with or in advance of an army or regiment, having spades, pickaxes, etc. to dig trenches, repair roads, and perform other labours in clearing and preparing the way for the main body." Armed with their international guidelines, these trial pioneers advanced their work in the morass of private-sector science, globalization, and state reform, and in the process they were stitching together a new public/private matrix that could facilitate experimentality.

But Dr. Mazur also introduced me to the "negative" characters, people he felt were "too opportunistic." Focused on immediate returns, these people did not play according to the power structures and norms of the enterprise. As one of his lawyer-colleagues told me later that week, "Investigators are supposed to be passive instruments." Throughout my work, I heard many stories about "overeager" investigators who refused to be passive instruments of research or who overenrolled patients for treatment purposes or for financial profit. I found this term quite curious, and I wondered whether its use was meant to help me appreciate the cultural crudeness from which Dr. Mazur (and others) must try to eke out professional expertise.

AR/CH had recently contracted with hypertension specialist Dr. Kamin-ska (a pseudonym), who had for two decades worked at a state-run medical center and its outpatient clinic. With a colleague, she had recently opened a private clinical trials office in the center's immediate vicinity. She recruited patients from the center for industry-sponsored trials (related to the treat-ment of chronic diseases such as hypertension and metabolic disorders such as diabetes and obesity) that she coordinated from her office. In the outpa-tient clinic of the medical center, she identified potential trial subjects who, given the high demand on the center's services, "had to wait a long time in the public health system to get examinations and treatments or could not afford to get them privately." While she could attract many volunteers—"I get two new patients a day," she told me—she was one of the overeager in-vestigators Dr. Mazur remained wary of.

I met Dr. Kaminska at her office not long after I had spoken with Dr. Mazur. It was early morning, and several volunteers had been sitting along a bench in a corridor, awaiting examination. Her phone was ringing off the hook because she had given patients "permission to call me any time of the day if they have any complaints or concerns. . . . I have a group of fif-teen long-term patients whom I treat. They keep asking, 'Do you have an-other research program for me?'" Dr. Kaminska was particularly skilled at enticing "stubborn patients with diet and lifestyle problems, as well as be-havioral and compliance issues" into research. Her work, as she suggested, was as much about research as it was about getting patients to take new medications. "I also have patients who don't want to take medicines," she told me. "They say they just want to be on a good diet. Then I say to them, 'I have a research program, let's see whose theory is right.' We get more de-tails about a patient's health and, in the end, we both win."

Dr. Kaminska described herself as very interested in research but noted that state science is vastly underfunded. Also, it takes a long time, she said, to master a given trial protocol—"It is a lot of work"—and she resented the fact that the number of patients allocated to her part of the study was "so small." She wanted to interpret her own data; she rejected the idea that any investigators who take part in a multinational study "cannot really have access to their own data in isolation because their sample is too small," as Dr. Mazur put it. Dr. Kaminska didn't think of herself as a passive techni-cian and strove to capitalize on her recruitment opportunities and control data. When she turned to the subject of monitoring, it became clear why Dr. Kaminska was potentially untamable. She said that the trial monitors who visited her from AR/CH weekly were more of a problem than a help:

"They are too young and they want to be too smart. In fact, they should just be a medium of communication." Dr. Kaminska was not interested in becoming an instrument for others. "I want to enroll more patients in my trials, not just a few." In spite of her prodigious enrollment talents and enthusiasm, AR/CH dropped her as a paid investigator.

Dr. Mazur's colleagues opened up to me. They told me how their branch of the globalized trial became a thriving enterprise, the problems they faced, and the professional identities they forged. To counterbalance this entrepreneurial account, I also spoke with academic scientists and state regulators and monitors in the country's FDA-equivalent body.[29] These actors did not fully endorse the industry's promotion of clinical trials as social goods, and they invariably invoked the need for a stronger state presence in both research oversight and public health policy. Their views expanded my interest in the varied levels of protection and risk that mark offshored research.

Dr. Zygmunt Sadovsky,[30] the acclaimed founder and first chairman of the Polish National Institute of Cardiology, made a Polish translation of the Good Clinical Practice standards. A Warsaw native, the good-humored seventy-year-old academician/scientist is now retired. We met that June at his office at the institute, away from the frantic bustle of young cardiologists and nurses and the intense flow of patients. I wanted to interview him, as he had played a key role in promoting international clinical research at his institute and in Poland. The author of more than three hundred published articles, "sixty in good international journals," he told me, Dr. Sadovsky traveled widely and had many contacts in the world of cardiology research. In the early nineties, he was vice-chair of the Polish drug regulatory agency. I was curious to learn his thoughts about issues of medical authority and ethics, now that trials had become so pervasive in cardiology- and oncology-related public health services. Industry estimates, for example, indicate that roughly 30 percent of expenditures on oncological treatment in Polish hospitals is covered as part of a clinical trials program.[31] Indeed, as Dr. Mazur told me, this and other medical fields were "awash" in experimental therapies.

Initially, Dr. Sadovsky and I talked about the Chernobyl nuclear disaster, as he wanted to know more about my prior anthropological work. "Chernobyl was a real experiment, a real disaster," he seconded my brief account. He then began to talk about the "cardiological disaster" that Poland faced in the 1980s and 1990s and that he helped to remediate: "We had a cardiovascular disease disaster. Fifty-two point seven percent of all adults were dying from it. We had one of the highest mortality rates due to acute myocardial infarction [heart attack] in the world. Our public health service was totally unprepared to fight this disaster." Dr. Sadovsky traced the crisis to poor nutrition, saturated fat, and other lifestyle factors such as smoking and alcohol consumption—all related to post–World War II and communist-era internal migration patterns and overall sociopolitical stress.

In the mid-1980s, while conducting his own research on various cardiovascular drugs (mainly thrombolytics, or clot-busting drugs), Dr. Sadovsky was contacted by a National Institutes of Health officer. This occasioned an "epidemiological exchange": "They were interested in the epidemiology of cardiovascular disease, and they wanted to know how bad it was in Poland. So I made my rounds across America in the eighties and early nineties." The international collaborations that ensued opened a space for the "disaster" to be publicly recognized. Soon a world-renowned cardiologist based at a prestigious American university contacted Dr. Sadovsky and asked him to participate in what were known as the GUSTO trials (large-scale trials of thrombolytic therapy for acute myocardial infarction). Poland was the ideal site because, as Dr. Sadovsky noted, Western European doctors were using cardiac intervention (catheterization) as the standard of care, whereas Polish doctors still relied on thrombolytics (intravenous medicines). That meant that Poles would willingly enroll in trials that included thrombolytic therapies as a comparison. All five GUSTO trials enrolled more than 200,000 patients internationally. Dr. Sadovsky coordinated the Polish sites. "These were the world's first megatrials."

In providing this background, Dr. Sadovsky was placing Poland's present trial bonanza in historical perspective, and he was conveying his critical judgment of where clinical research had strayed from legitimate public health concerns. "We didn't start from zero," he told me. "We had a really good start with GUSTO 1."

"Why were you invited to participate in these studies?" I asked.

"Then and now, in the United States there are many rules and it is not easy to recruit patients. Rules—this is part of why the GUSTO studies went international. Moreover, our American colleagues looked for competent technicians who could execute the studies. We had substantial input in this trial because of the large number of patients we recruited and because we had very good documentation in English. The organizers were quite surprised."

Dr. Sadovsky was proud to have participated in trials that set the standard for cardiac care internationally. They gave him epidemiological know-how and scientific capital in Solidarity-era Poland. But what he savored most was his own academic contribution to the public health efforts that he was able to champion. The Polish National Institute of Cardiology's hospital facility, which had been underutilized, was made available to the general public: "The worst cases were transferred here from all over Poland and all the beds were filled." Dr. Sadovsky was also a driving force behind a nationwide cardiovascular risk-prevention effort from 1992 to 2001. The initiative led to a significant drop in cardiovascular mortality in 2001—a kind of health transition at warp speed.

With new diagnostic technologies and treatment possibilities available, and with strong governmental support, Dr. Sadovsky and colleagues were able to significantly enhance Poland's cardiac care infrastructure. "Since 1993, we added sixty new CAT labs in Poland." He compared the state of cardiac care in Poland with that of his former communist neighbor to the east. "The Ukrainian city of Lviv, for example, has no CAT labs. Now we have four CAT labs, just in our institute!" More people could be assessed for surgical interventions, and this in turn created new platforms for cardiology research.

Given Dr. Sadovsky's success, researchers from other American universities asked him to coordinate Polish centers for riskier multinational trials of surgical treatments for ischemic heart failures such as the ISIS 2 and STICH trials. These were not simple trials by any stretch. The latter involved complicated procedures such as open-heart surgery, coronary artery bypass graft surgery, and surgical ventricular restoration. The logistical complexity of such multicentered trials was also staggering. It was necessary to coordinate information regarding thousands of heart attack patients in different countries who, within twenty-four hours of onset of a suspected heart attack and hospitalization, had to give their informed consent and be randomized. The chief of the institute's intensive care unit told me about the difficulties of enrolling patients: "Many patients are in shock when they are hospitalized. Getting informed consent from family members is too complicated. Our laws say to go to a judge and ask for permission, but that takes too much time. We prefer to wait for the moment when the person comes out of shock, and that is when we get the consent."

The institute's recruitment capacity, high ethical standards, and technical excellence had opened the door to globalized trials in Poland. Yet Dr. Sadovsky set and maintained very strict criteria regarding the trials in which the institute would participate. He refused to be a cog in the "industrialization" of trials and closed the door on projects that he believed had little scientific and public health merit. "Both sides must be able to obtain *relevant* knowledge," he told me, measured in terms of the success of clinical outcomes. "We need real progress here, as we had in the reduction of cardiovascular mortality rates."

By the time Dr. Mazur joined the trial scene, the institute was off-limits, both because it was inundated with trials and because it had become highly selective of the trials it accepted. Professionals who worked at the institute and had spun off private medical offices began to be pursued as investigators. Other medical facilities that had been overshadowed by the powerful institute now had the chance to profit from the trial enterprise as well. They are able to recruit high numbers of patients but, unlike the institute, these less prestigious sites' negotiating power with companies is limited, as are the benefits that they are able to channel for enrolled patients.

I spoke to a busy, middle-aged cardiologist, trained in Poland and in the United States in intervention cardiology. He worked in what he called one of the institute's "competitor sites," located in one of Warsaw's poorest boroughs. "Industry can't recruit at the institute anymore, so they started coming to us," Dr. Jasiński (a pseudonym) told me as we sat in his office. We were surrounded by white veneer furniture bearing the clean, sweeping lines typical of Herman Miller office furniture. Everything was new—office equipment, CAT lab and computers, file cabinets and desk and chairs—"all paid for by the industry." I couldn't help but notice a dented gray desk lamp. This, Dr. Jasiński explained, he kept as a kind of souvenir of old, aesthetically drab communist times. "We have really bad untreated chronic diseases here," he said, and then added, sarcastically, "It's a gold mine."

Poland's cardiac medical culture and efficient interventions, according to Dr. Jasiński, make for an excellent clinical trials environment. "In our hospitals, there is better interaction among cardiologists who do the diagnostic assessments and cardiac surgeons who do the interventions. And 'door-to-needle time' is much shorter."[32] Dr. Jasiński argued that the American medical culture is "too litigious." The admission, diagnostic, and intervention process is fragmented and overly specialized, and bureaucracy limits both recruitment and patient survival prospects: "From initial assessment to the operating room, it can take at least four hours." Dr. Jasiński handed me an article he had written showing that standard informed consent procedures—if followed to the letter—significantly and dangerously added to the "door-to-needle time." It was evident that his specialty was not just cardiological intervention but also the recruitment of acute heart attack patients into clinical research. He did not question his own problematic interpretation of informed consent as basically a time-consuming matter.

Another problem, according to Dr. Jasiński, is that "American doctors are overpaid, and they are on call and not in the clinic. We get no money, so we stay here day and night—older and younger colleagues alike. It couldn't be a more different system." In Dr. Jasiński 's hospital, the door-to-needle time amounts to about twenty minutes. "We have Admissions just one floor below my office. I just go down and in five minutes the patient is in here, right in the CAT lab. There isn't any more bureaucracy. If I see that a patient should have surgery, I do it immediately, or I contact another skilled surgeon."

According to Dr. Jasiński, Poland's higher patient recruitment for cardiological interventions reflects not simply a public health crisis and "exploitation," but the fact that Poland has the technical capacity to save lives and also to recruit these patients for clinical research. Here, the notion that drug companies or CROs need substandard regulatory environments and unscrupulous physicians in order to institutionalize their research globally is not true. Indeed, cardiology trial recruitment involves split-second decision making and is full of gray zones, wherever it takes place. Dr. Jasiński conceded that "a lot of mistakes and misjudgments can happen" in patient recruitment. But he also felt that Poland's good medical organization and timely emergency response offered more patient protection than informed consent per se. In his rendering, quality care trumps ethical procedure. But Dr. Jasiński did not further elaborate on this experimentality that is now part and parcel of medical care.[33]

Akademia Kliniczna

June 20, 2005. I was wending my way through the cobblestoned streets of the Old City quarters of Sławen, located four hours by train from Warsaw, and situated in the sprawling rural fields of southeast Poland, not far from the Ukrainian border. With a population of 360,000, Sławen is one of the largest cities in the region. There are ten hospitals in the city proper, three of which are affiliated with Sławen's medical academy, and five more in nearby towns.

The Old City's structures, built in the fifteenth century and rebuilt many times since, have been recently renovated. In dark archways, mounted plaques recount a long history of harmony among Jews, Christians, and Muslims. The stark realities of World War II belie such portrayals. The Nazis desecrated Sławen's Jewish community and its cultural patrimony. Several kilometers away from the town center is the site of a notorious concentration camp, where 78,000 people, mainly Jews, were killed.

I was in Sławen to meet a former medical school administrator, whom I shall refer to as Dr. Turek, and who, in Dr. Mazur's words, was a "clinical trials pioneer." A specialist in internal medicine, Dr. Turek had, since 1993, conducted dozens of industry-sponsored trials. Educated in Warsaw, he trained several generations of doctors and placed them in the region's medical institutions. He had recently established a clinic/freestanding research facility with colleagues and former students. The facility conducts trials in more than a dozen medical subdisciplines. I noticed several pharmacies along the way with big white signs posted above their doorways. They read "Akademia Kliniczna" with arrows pointing toward the facility. I followed them. It was almost 2:00 p.m., the time Dr. Turek expected me in his office. A nurse took me past the patient waiting area and monitoring rooms to an end-of-the corridor office space. There, Dr. Turek, a genteel, English-speaking, quick-witted senior man, greeted me effusively. The high ceilings and plastered rococo details of his office were painted pure white. The beige leather sofas were set upon richly colored carpets. Arrangements of freshly cut flowers filled vases. A nurse handed us delicate porcelain cups filled with tea drawn from a samovar. Each element was an echo of the style of the Polish colonial nobility once situated along the country's easternmost border. As nurses walked in and out of Dr. Turek's office, patients sat in adjacent rooms, craning to catch glimpses of the nearby luxury.

Dr. Turek started a second career in clinical research in the early nineties, when he was asked to take part in a multisited trial for a major-selling prescription drug. The drug belonged to a class of new antacids—proton pump inhibitors—already being marketed in the United States and Western Europe. These were the days of the "antacid wars" (Goozner 2004:219). Companies were competing for a piece of the $7-billion-a-year market in antacids.[34] They sponsored hundreds of me-too drug trials, eager to show the benefit of their antacid brand over other brands.

Dr. Turek explained that this particular me-too drug trial was also a rescue study. To prove the drug's efficacy in stopping or stemming ulceration, the trial required patients who were being treated for rheumatoid arthritis. The older class of rheumatoid arthritis drugs—known as nonsteroidal anti-inflammatory drugs (NSAIDs)—damage the stomach and can create ulcers. Patient inclusion criteria called for patients who were using NSAIDs, but who had no prior history of proton pump inhibitor use. Additionally, patients had to have previously undiagnosed ulcers identified by invasive gastroscopies. We have heard this story before: with a "gamed" cohort, the trial's goal of proving the new drug's effectiveness could be more easily achieved. A year into the trial, Western European investigators had not been able to

meet their recruitment goals, partly because most Western European patients were already on proton pump inhibitors. Running behind schedule,
the trial's sponsor turned to a noted American trial entrepreneur who, in
turn, dispatched a clinical research associate to Poland. She found help in
Dr. Turek.

Finding patients was easy, this physician said: "I worked in one of the region's main and much-sought-after university hospitals. We saw almost two
million patients per year there as well as in various internal medicine wards
in regional hospitals. I visited all of the wards and asked physicians to identify patients with certain symptoms. Many of the physicians were former
students of mine. I told them that I could offer patients a new drug or a
placebo, and that gastroscopies would be free of charge. They began to send
me their patients. They continue to send patients here."

With a sort of giddy pride, Dr. Turek told me that although he had been
given only two months, through a marathon of gastroscopies he was able to
identify forty-one trial subjects with new ulcers. "The Western European investigators had one year and could not find that many patients." He ended
up being one of the trial's top two recruiters. "We came in second, but we
had such a short recruitment time!" The drug manufacturer rewarded the
principal investigators of the three highest recruitment centers with first authorship in a top medical journal, Dr. Turek explained. In industry circles,
he was recognized as a clinical trials hero of sorts. "They asked me, 'Dr.
Turek, how much money do you want to run a trial?' And I always replied,
'As much as you can give me.'"

One study monitor at AR/CH told me that the Sławen site played a crucial role in the company's operations. "We have ninety gastroenterological
and arthritis patients in this site." Seen from this on-the-ground perspective, patients are valued less for a supposed treatment naïveté and more for
their learned experimental behavior. "Most of them participated in some
other clinical trial before they participated in a recent one sponsored by us."
Almost all of Dr. Turek's regular patients had participated in a clinical trial,
he told me, and after a drug "wash-out" period, they enrolled in new trials
if they were eligible. Serial enrollers were considered more reliable and compliant than first-time subjects.

Perhaps sensing my concerns over ethics in this study mill, Dr. Turek assured me that his patients participated in his trials "voluntarily." He then
told me about a patient who, he said, "was so committed" to the research
process that he could not say no. "This patient was highly educated, an
engineer, and participated in a trial for a nonsteroidal anti-inflammatory

drug. I always reassured him that he could quit at any time, and that he wouldn't lose his medical care. One day he came to me with his weekly gastroscopy results in hand and said, 'Doctor, I have a real problem. I thought that I could participate in the entire trial.' He enumerated all the lesions [ulcers] and hemorrhoids the gastroscopy had revealed. After that, he told me, 'Now I have a *legitimate* reason to stop—not by my own choice, but because the protocol dictates so.'" Dr. Turek intended this story to be an illustration of the depth of his patients' commitment to the trial process. But to me, it conveyed a rather different point: arguably, only through injury could this patient feel free to leave the trial. And, even as he was dropping out, he wanted to protect his access to specialized care in the future. Dr. Turek did not say whether this patient's ulcers were study related. Only the patient would know.

Since he had clinical experience with nonsteroidal anti-inflammatory drugs, I asked Dr. Turek what he thought of the postmarketing evidence of cardiovascular risk associated with one popular anti-inflammatory drug and the drug's subsequent withdrawal from the market. He said that he had run trials for the drug, but quickly added, "I don't feel guilty about it." He offered an elaborate explanation that focused on the drug's dangerous biochemical mechanisms that he believed should have been evident to the manufacturer before human trials began. But then, he insisted, "without clinical trials, we would never know which medicine is safe." He said that trial subjects "are necessary to medical progress." The investigator himself is not to be blamed for undertaking a dangerous trial, and, as if to shift the burden of responsibility of deciphering risks onto patients, he added, "They come knowing that this is a risky enterprise." Moreover, "the industry has considerably improved trial safety." The trials of the anti-inflammatory drug in question, Dr. Turek stipulated, "took place in Poland *pre*-ICH-GCP. Things were a lot riskier then." Regulation tames problematic trial safety, but the power differentials that afforded careless medical practice remain intact.

The Work of Slack

In order to conform to new global trade rules, countries had to establish new regulatory bodies, mandate ethical review boards, and support a culture of ethics and accountability. Poland had accepted ICH-GCP guidelines in 1997, when it passed a law on medical experimentation. Such delay in implementation is not by any stretch peculiar to Poland; it pertains to other countries in the region and to other world regions as well.[35] But as a local pharmaceutical industry lawyer told me, this law has been enforced "mainly since 2002." Until 2002, "bureaucracy was minimal," a Polish drug regulatory official told me. "Trials commenced regardless of whether local ethics committees were in place. If a hospital director wanted a trial, he could start it. No problem. There was no delay. No national system of regulation or clinical trials registration was in place."

Insights from Albert O. Hirschman's classic *Exit, Voice, and Loyalty* can help us to better understand the productiveness of such regulatory lag periods when competitiveness can be maximized. Hirschman's book focuses on the decline of firms and states and on their organizational responses. For him, the image of the economy as a fully competitive system is a "defective representation." He dismisses the idea that "changes in the fortunes of individual firms are exclusively caused by basic shifts of comparative advantage" and argues that the criteria of best performance are indeed "murky" (1970:2). Hirschman's insights also prompt interesting questions about how drug development outsourcing can become a defensive strategy by threatened producers and sponsors.[36] In the actual world, Hirschman argues, the fortunes of firms and states are intimately linked to the handling of "more or less permanent pockets of inefficiency and neglect"—or "slack." Human societies and economic organizations "have a wide latitude for deterioration" and develop "mechanisms of recuperation," such as exit and voice.

Hirschman sees firms and states as permanently and randomly subject to decline and decay, "that is, to a gradual loss of rationality, efficiency, and surplus-producing energy, no matter how well the institutional framework within which they function is designed." Moreover, "it is likely that the very process of decline activates certain counterforces" (ibid.:15). Professionals in the clinical trials industry speak disarmingly about the inefficiencies and failures that are built into drug development, and about themselves as a counterforce of decline (see chapter 2). This sense of decline is widely touted. In the words of Hein Besselaar, "Of 10,000 chemical compounds only 100 are tested in animals. Of those 100, 10 go into human testing and 1 becomes a marketable drug. The 9,999 potential drugs that fall by the wayside have cost some money somewhere. A lot of money is wasted."

The series of numbers—10,000, 100, 10, 1—marks a reality of diminishing returns. And Dr. Besselaar suggested that beneath the dearth of products lay vast opportunities for recuperative work. The CRO professionals I spoke to saw themselves, in part, as the remediators of a business model that had, from a scientific and practical standpoint, "gone bust." But economically, that model had a peculiar life of its own. New competitive clinical trials environments are constantly being tailored to test drugs and bring them to the market rapidly.[37] Trial sponsors need unexplored territories, pivotal countries, and "reserve" or rescue countries to root experimentality to sustain a predominant business model and to offset its diminishing returns. The "massive arbitrage" that "is really the definition of globalisation" (Garnier 2005:2) remedies declines in productivity by supplying endless laboratories for the sake of the (drug approval) experiment. Sponsors to some extent rely on outside actors to resolve the paradoxes of their business model, and this is where the work of CROs seems to matter most.

But to the extent that the object of experimentality is also there to support "pseudo filings in the patent law, me-too drugs, and product indication extensions," that object is far from being value-neutral or devoid of social and political nuance. My CRO interlocutors were in a constant fix over having to make personal judgment calls, choosing between alternatives that were not obviously right or wrong. They rarely spoke about any specific transgression but, rather, about systemic flaws. Slack created its own effervescence— ever more specialized niches for other business entities to enter into the clinical trial chain. In the process, responsibility for dangerous protocols, for example, could be deferred. The risks attached to this sort of deferral can apparently go unconsidered, at least for some (profitable) time period. Most of the professionals I knew remained loyal (and competitive) within a flawed system rather than exercising "voice." They campaigned for optimal regulatory combinations and relied on an array of medical and social collaborators for their success, without threatening the overall system. In a way, they were their sponsors' best defense, insofar as it was their job to "monitor" experimentality and purge it of any political content—to make it an alternative form of health care in ailing local medical institutions. The idea of slack illustrates well how the globalized clinical trial becomes such a successful public/private enterprise, and how its workings become a political matter or, rather, are prevented from becoming one.[38] Experimentality requires wide latitudes of deterioration (to use Hirschman's term) to be cost-effective. But whose job is it to pick up the slack that experimentality leaves behind?

Dr. Mazur spoke disparagingly about Poland before good clinical practice standards were in place—the "pre-ICH-GCP period"—when it was used "as a rescue country. Now we have very high ethical standards." Playing the rescue role for the drug industry was certainly not unique to Poland; this positioning as reserved territory for foreign trial sponsors often reflects an earlier moment in a country's trial market expansion. His American counterpart, Dr. Francis, explained to me how projects that failed to produce a marketable product or that lost commercial interest were often "dumped." Researchers in nascent trial destination countries were charged with "salvaging" the study drug, that is, studying its effectiveness in another proposed application or actually searching for new uses for it. Dumping was common in Latin America, she said. "If the companies aren't going to make more money on a drug, they may pass it to the local corporate affiliate. They just pass it along." When a new drug or drug class begins to dominate a market, the demand for the old drug wanes. But the research cycle for the old drug often continues in the form of salvage-type research—and that is where "dumping" becomes a potentially profitable form of rescue.

I had first heard about this salvage-type research from a Brazilian physician who was part of her country's nascent clinical trials industry in the early 1990s. Dr. Santos (a pseudonym), a former director of clinical research in cardiac and psychiatric drug development for a leading multinational corporation with an affiliate in Brazil, was trained in Brazil and completed a medical residency in Canada. I had heard about her from other medical colleagues in the southern city of Porto Alegre. Dr. Santos was now working in a local medical rehabilitation facility, and she happily agreed to talk to me about that time in her life that was "now over."

In the early 1990s, Brazil was *terra nova* for international clinical research, Dr. Santos told me. "It was not saturated with trials." As a clinical research director, Dr. Santos coordinated her company's trials and recruited prominent clinical investigators in cardiology and psychiatry, particularly key opinion leaders who were willing to evaluate products in accordance with her company's marketing aims. She also audited her company's investigator sites in Brazil and in Western Europe. After having achieved financial stability, Dr. Santos left the industry—"I wanted to be able to sleep at night."

Dr. Santos had seen drug development from the "other side," as she put it. Echoing Dr. Francis's depiction of the dumping process, she managed projects that were passed along from the North either because drugs failed on the market and had to be given a new destiny, or because projects had been left behind by highly mobile medical directors "who had moved to other posts in other parts of the world":

All of us had to answer to medical directors in each specialty who were mostly foreigners. My boss was a Norwegian—a very nice person who did not know Portuguese and knew nothing of Brazilian culture and poverty. She was here and, like others in her position, was already looking four or five years ahead in her career, one step higher, a different country, a more promising trial. Whereas we [the nationals] were looking at the budget and targeting the budget to win money. This was our focus.

Salvaging old drugs dominated Dr. Santos's workload: "Unfortunately, there were a lot of errors with the new drugs entering the market. I had to work *inside* the mistakes," she emphasized. Dr. Santos told me the story of an antibiotic that had been very successful in the European market, but the launch had failed in Brazil—"it did not kill any bacteria." In her salvage work, Dr. Santos discovered contributing factors rooted in climate and economic differences. "Many people here lacked refrigerators to store the drug," and, just as importantly, "populations that we tested were undernourished and had no protein to link the drug." Her work led to a different chemical formulation and eventually to a relaunching of the drug in Latin America.

A more typical case of "working inside the mistake" involved the reengineering of a new antidepressant. "A drug was launched into the market at 150 milligrams daily." But, in the postmarketing phase, questions arose about the effectiveness of the drug. The company turned to Dr. Santos to quickly recruit patients and rerun a Phase 3 trial. Time was of the essence. Trials were easier to launch in Brazil at that time, she explained, as there were no hindering regulations and a good medical infrastructure was in place. "I could immediately contact prominent Brazilian psychiatrists who were on the company's payroll and were opinion makers. They worked in eight major university hospitals across the country and could rapidly recruit from outpatient wards."

Trial results indicated that the drug didn't work, "a placebo, sugar in water." Dr. Santos's team then mixed small doses of a powerful hypnotic drug with this antidepressant and had plans to relaunch the new combined drug at double the original recommended dose. Coincidentally, a Brazilian law prohibiting such combined drug formulations had just come into effect. "Thank God!" Dr. Santos exclaimed, happy that this timely law had stopped her from carrying out the practices she now deemed "unethical."

With or without the added hypnotic, Dr. Santos remained unconvinced of the ability of the drug's higher dose formulation to treat major depression. So she "looked for another illness that the failed drug could work for." In the end, her medical and marketing teams were able to place the drug (which has never received FDA approval) on the Brazilian market for the treatment of a mild form of depression—a "made-up" illness, as she called it. As Dr. Santos clarified, "Sometimes working inside the mistake meant working inside the illness. It was a money machine."

Dr. Santos's experiences in Brazil, like those of Dr. Turek in Poland, point to a set of offshored environments that can be activated at a moment's notice to deal with drug-development slack, augmenting patient enrollment or remedying scientific and postmarketing errors. Their research was ethical according to the given standards. Dr. Santos described the ethics informing her company's local practices as "very idealistic and legalistic," while also noting that "many patients signed informed consent documents with their fingerprints." In retrospect and in comparative perspective, salvage research operates and relocates according to a logic of circumvention and opportunity. Yet the document-driven ethics that legitimates it is dependent on the immediate interests and morality of the individuals involved in running the trials. In this recycling machine of clinical trials, it is entirely possible to be ethically compliant yet "still fail to be ethical," as Dr. Santos put it. On top of that, she was willing to admit her complicity in a dangerous science; external safeguards to this kind of research are sporadic at best.

Patient-Consumers

Critics of the growth of clinical trials in developing countries have pointed to subject coercion, the lack of voluntary and informed participation, and inadequately informed consent as the most common problems. Industry actors and some medics, on the other hand, tend to promote clinical trials as a social good in medically or materially impoverished contexts. They emphasize the access participation provides to otherwise unavailable treatments and individuals' willingness to participate, casting subjects as patient-consumers.[39] But, as I have been showing in this chapter, the language of coercion or of rational choice does not fully capture the multiple conditions that make experimental scenarios possible. Reworking ideas of patienthood and care is central to this experimentality. Recall Dr. Santos's story of the fingerprinted informed consent or Dr. Turek's "so committed" subject who could not say no.

Henryk Król (a pseudonym) works for a firm specializing in patient re-cruitment. He gave me insights into how pharmaceutical ideas of consumer-patienthood drive recruitment, while rendering concerns over subject coer-cion moot. These practices raise questions about the integrity of the informed consent process and remain underproblematized in traditional discourses of patient rights and medical malpractice. Król, whom I met in Poland in 2005, leads his firm's expansion in Eastern Europe and oversees the activities of clinical trial monitors. Very polite and austere, Król was known for his pinpoint accuracy in identifying and fixing potential errors in the clinical trials documentation process.

At one point during our discussions, he offered an example of an "enter-prising" recruitment strategy. The story was about how to enlist untreated patients for a placebo-controlled study, but to do so in an ethical way. He thought the approach was brilliant. I found it disturbing. Here is the se-quence of operations: "We all know that it is unethical to withdraw treat-ment from patients during a trial. If patients can get the required treatment where they live, then we certainly cannot withhold treatment or use a placebo," he said. "Whereas for a patient with a newly diagnosed condition, say hypertension, withholding treatment is ethically justified."

"How so?" I asked.

"You cannot put the second patient immediately on the medication any-way. It is totally acceptable to wait and see if, say, the patient's hypertension can be controlled by nonpharmaceutical means." A patient can be treated "through diet, less salt, exercise," Król added.

What was disturbing here was that this lifestyle treatment approach was simply a stepping-stone to turning this patient into a placebo subject. In this instance, a recruiter's task is to identify people who are in a "window" of nontreatment. But that window, as Król hints, must be engineered. He illus-trated his point with an example: "Say you are an investigator. You go to a factory with people doing a stressful lifting kind of work. You tell the work-ers, 'We are doing research on cholesteremia [high cholesterol levels], which may indicate hypertension or diabetes, and we want to examine your lipid levels. If your level is higher, we might offer you this study drug.'" Król was quick to add that the investigator was doing the workers a favor, that is, offering them a diagnostic gift: "The workers would have never known that they have a health problem otherwise. They may not even be familiar with the names of these diseases."

At this stage, information is offered as a means of drumming up people's interest in trial participation. Once willing to enter the trial, Król said,

"They will learn about the treatment. They will also learn that these drugs are quite expensive, twenty to thirty dollars a month for two packs of lipid-lowering treatments." Then, he said, "*They are now fully informed* and can enter the trial." In his account, informed consent happens once potential patient-consumers understand the high cost of a drug—well before they enter a trial. The prospect of having free access to high-priced drugs and frequent medical supervision incites their willingness to be on a placebo arm, he reasons. In Król's account, the investigator cleverly plays up the placebo-arm as a possible stepping-stone to bigger and better things, but we will never know the full scope of the manipulation of expectations on the ground. "When these workers enter a placebo-control trial, they know there's a fifty-fifty chance that they will get the treatment. They also know they will be seen every two weeks instead of every six months. Their lab tests will be performed in one of our Western European laboratories."

The recruitment process in this instance merges with the creation of a patient-consumer who buys into a particular idea of disease, who is educated by the trial recruiter about the best possible treatment, and who realizes that he is unable to get that care outside of a trial. *The moment of buy-in is the moment of informed consent.* Consent in this case has been culturally reoriented toward the pharmaceutical and toward a consumer-patienthood that is yet to be fulfilled. And this is quite different from the traditional informed consent, in which personal autonomy is somehow maintained. This is not exactly coercion either, as it blends with the offer of medical goods (care, drugs, lab work, etc.). Potential trial subjects in this corporate rendition of consent are not vulnerable or poor, but free agents. To choose not to participate in the trial would constitute a lost opportunity.[40]

Król's ethics—couched in today's universal terms, "We all know that it is unethical to withdraw treatment from patients during a trial"—is primarily retooled as an instrument of recruitment rather than as an instrument of protection. A certain scientific rigor that is so highly valorized in the clinical trials process appears to be untarnished, and coercion is seemingly not an issue yet. For Król, the moment of informed consent is the moment when the patient is fully informed *and* exposed to the pharmaceutical market and its limited mechanisms of access. Reading between the lines, there is a vague threat of withholding treatment unless a patient joins a study, but no one is making that threat. For many, experiments have become the only mechanism of access. This moment of "exposure" is nowhere to be documented. In Król's example, no party finds the use of the placebo to be unethical, no one has performed a socially bad action, and there is no transgression to be redressed. Yet it also shows how informed consent is one moment in an intricate game of profit and loss. The long and intriguing process through which a person comes to "voluntarily" consent to participating in a trial is not easily observed in this ethical transparency.

"Our society was not competitive"

Dr. Mazur put me in contact with another of his colleagues, this time an individual from the Czech Republic. I met the head of Tem/po's clinical trials operations in the Czech Republic in late 2005 when he came to the United States to attend a business meeting at the company's headquarters. In his fifties, this former Czech public health worker, whom I will call Martin, had fifteen years of business experience, earning him a quiet and relaxed self-confidence. "In a nutshell, how would you describe your work?" I asked him. "I transform the market," he told me.

Over the course of our two-hour conversation, it became obvious to me that Martin was a seasoned player in the "big game of clinical trials." He calls forth and enlists resources that are either scattered or badly utilized in health-care environments and turns them into what he referred to as "competitive environments." Gesturing as if he were moving chess pieces, Martin said, "Here's the academic research site. Over here is the neighborhood polyclinic. If there is an academic site that we want to attract but that is too slow to join, we say to them, 'Look over here. Here is a [nonacademic] polyclinic—look how well it is doing.' Otherwise they won't move."

Born in the industrial city of Brno, Martin received his medical training at the country's most venerable university and throughout the 1980s worked as a chemist in Czech public health institutions. In the early 1990s, he studied epidemiology in the United Kingdom. "I became familiar with the randomized control trial"—a technique that, as he put it, was generally not known or practiced by Eastern European or Soviet investigators. He also trained in disease control programs in the United States. Martin described himself as part of a "wave of Czech experts" who brought their new know-how back home. They sought professional mobility in newly established pharmaceutical subsidiaries.

Martin spoke of the pharmaceutical industry's presence as an indicator of his country's move from political collapse to economic competitiveness. "There was a quiet and chaotic transition at all levels of society, including the public health service and its privatization, restructuring, and of course, research. State-governed research had collapsed. Of course, I am not saying everything was bad, just that our society was not competitive." A regulatory void was crucial in providing a foothold for this emergent competitiveness, and Martin clearly took advantage of the institutionalized slack. Indeed, he viewed his entrepreneurial know-how as integral to the state-building capacity of the Czech Republic:

> There was no Good Clinical Practice guideline, no International Conference on Harmonisation, nothing. Between 1990 and 1995, when larger companies arrived in Central-Eastern Europe, there were no regulatory affairs offices, no capacities in the Ministries of Health. The mentality of policy makers was different than it is now. Their population thinking was totally different. I would say that the early to mid-1990s marked our pioneer period, like the Klondike [gold rush] period in America. I was probably one of the first to arrive from abroad as a clinical research associate and consultant for a pharmaceutical company affiliate. Then I joined another firm in the mid-1990s. I brought software and technical things, like remote data entry systems, to the Czech Republic, Russia, and elsewhere. There was no infrastructure, or it was not working.

This minimalistic clinical trials environment was made functional and cost-effective, mainly because it was attached to an ailing but still functional universal public health-care system. "For companies it was cheap; they got good data quick. There was a need for services, and all of a sudden Western companies realized the huge potential here. There was an extremely good population pool in terms of medical indicators, both chronic and acute diseases. The population was not treated by remedies that were available in the West, so it was quite attractive. There were treatment-naive, steroid-naive, statin-naive people—people you could hardly find in the U.S. or Western Europe. We had extremely high recruitment rates."

Like Poland, the Czech Republic initially found its place in the globalized trial network as a rescue country. "There were a lot of trials that started in the West and then were shifted to the East. Where recruitment periods of four months yielded zero patients in Western Europe, a two-week recruitment period in Central-Eastern Europe yielded forty patients. Arthritis and antibiotic studies were quite popular in the Czech Republic. Poland was the place to go for rescue studies in urology and asthma. For asthma, a lot of steroid-naive patients could be found. It was all quite good."

In countries like Poland and the Czech Republic, the new disease categories and medical commodities that came with clinical research did not require a hard sell. Again and again, I heard from these informants that second-world patient populations, afflicted by but often not treated for their chronic diseases, were eager to embrace the West and its drugs, with all this activity happening in a context of narrowed choices and a sense of extreme vulnerability. As Martin talked, I recalled the informal networks of exchange and selling that evolved around sample antidepressants in Ukraine, among the Chernobyl physicians and sufferers I had worked with. Once structurally weak, the Soviet physician became a powerful gatekeeper of pharmaceutical goods that he or she alone was entrusted to dangle before the weary post-Soviet welfare subject. Martin detailed the crucial role of key local experts in making trials happen against the background of corruption and an apparent regulatory ignorance:

> Trials were rather simple to launch in the early years. If a Western European drug company was involved, its research associates just drove across the border. They carried the experimental product to the investigational site in their cars and then drove back. There were no customs payments. No one cared about the contents of the investigations. There weren't any ethical committees on site. If there were any, members did not know what they were supposed to do. Ethical approval was a mere formality. Only one form of approval was required, the minister of health's signature, which was also very simple to get.

The life cycle of this experimental order was, however, predictably short. Martin broke it up into three distinct phases. First, he told me, there was "the opportune moment," the gold rush. The industry needed quick recruitment into clinical trials for diseases that "our populations suffered from, and that Soviet public health had neglected in its prioritizing of diseases of security, such as those stemming from radiological, chemical, and other mass-destruction items. There was very little clinical research. The reality of chronic diseases such as cardiovascular diseases was obscured." Most Czechs could barely afford new Western medications for chronic ailments that were entering the market, said Martin. The state was not willing or able to pay for them either.

This brings us to the second phase of the clinical trials life cycle—the peak moment—when experiments become a "normal part of health delivery," said Martin, and when "people no longer view trial participation in terms of being examined like rabbits." At this stage, clinical trials appear to absorb public health needs. The categories of research subject and biological citizen conflate. With the inflow of clinical trials programs and human and financial capital, governments foster a culture of regulation, compliance, monitoring, and auditing, however soft or simulated that culture might be, but with all its expected features of supporting commercial work.

Then, Martin said, a moment arrives when these markets "become exhausted." This is the third stage of the clinical trials life cycle.

"What are the symptoms of exhaustion?" I asked.

"Trials start to migrate eastward, to Ukraine, Russia, Uzbekistan, and Kazakhstan." There are too many companies competing for high-quality investigators, and they become "too choosy." By this he meant that investigators choose trials that match their research interests or that they begin to charge the equivalent of Western European prices for their expertise. Also, Martin added, "People simply leave the trials." In his view, trial subjects for the most part are only "temporarily loyal," and after a while they drop out, no longer seeing any immediate advantage in participating in trials. In its movement east, the trials industry leaves behind some citizens who are now primed as patient-consumers. But it does not necessarily alter the conditions that drove its profitability in the first place.

As an illustration of this phenomenon, Martin noted that pools of "steroid-free asthmatic children" in the Czech Republic "are starting to get exhausted a little." At the point of increased competitiveness for the right kind of patients, and when regulations start to be less flexible, "it simply becomes too expensive for us, just as in the U.S., Western Europe, and Canada." Prior to the deterioration of this experimental environment, and always thinking ahead, the research industry starts up sites elsewhere in the region. According to Martin, the Czech clinical trials market "has less than ten years left." In the end, the globalized clinical trial floats away, leaving behind historical inequalities and intensely convoluted public-private relations in the field of health.

Pivotal Countries

Worldwide, governments are the primary purchasers of drugs, and drug pricing is "a country-by-country affair," as one senior contract research organization executive told me in November 2005. Most countries—the United States is a powerful exception—exercise price control, and there is intense pharmaceutical lobbying in this field. Companies reward countries that facilitate research and sales with further investments. In 2004 Astra-Zeneca, for example, threatened to reduce its clinical research investments in Sweden unless the government continued to purchase one of its proton pump inhibitors. Sweden's Drug and Therapeutics Committee recommended cheaper off-patent drugs and told the company, "Health care doesn't need more me-too drugs." To which AstraZeneca's global drug-development executive replied, "Why should we spend $1.2 billion Euros on research in Sweden when this country doesn't appreciate the work of our 5,000 researchers?"[41] Leveraging capacity varies greatly by country. Most Eastern European countries lack a truly competitive generics industry and are tethered to restrictive global trade laws. They also lack health technology assessment programs that could better inform pharmaceutical policies.

This professional seemed to suggest that within these institutionalized absences of negotiating power, the industry sorts out a strategic cartography of where to carry out trials, particularly of blockbuster drugs. The sorting is not just about study cost-effectiveness: "Location of testing is crucial for us to get the right indication [reason to prescribe] for the drug." In choosing a particular study site or country in which to run a study, companies know how to get data they need to support the right indication. He explained, "We also want to ensure the highest precedent price for a drug. So there is usually an important regulatory approval strategy that goes along with developing the drug." Initial U.S. FDA approval for a given drug application allows companies to set the highest possible precedent price for their new drug (since there is no price regulation in the United States). When marketed globally, new drugs will "ideally" be sold on the basis of that highest precedent price. It is crucial for companies, however, to carefully orchestrate the subsequent filing of a drug's application outside the United States to maximize pricing in regional markets (strategically placed marketing studies can ensure maximum pricing). "File in the wrong country, get a precedent price set in a low-pricing country, and this sweeps across the region, and that is a disaster."

Some countries play a more pivotal role than others in this highest-precedent-price strategy. They are often referred to as "pivotal countries." I heard industry professionals use this expression when referring to countries that had learned, in exchange for research investments, not to rock the price negotiation boat, and that are capable of influencing their neighbors' policies. Martin, for example, helped to shape the Czech Republic's pivotal status. But in the late nineties, in the heat of debates over the ethics of placebo use, the Czech legislature banned the use of the placebo in clinical trials. As a result, companies moved their investments to neighboring Hungary and the Baltic states, where placebo use was allowed.

Martin told me he worked hard to reverse the effects of this antiplacebo legislation. He urged lawmakers to change their stance: "I told them that we would no longer be competitive with Hungary. We will lose many opportunities." Soon the Czech lawmakers repealed the law, and the industry returned, he told me. Back at his firm's U.S. headquarters, Martin's boss read the Czech incident as being relatively benign—it created an opportunity for other countries to compete. "You can shop around if the Czech Republic rejects you." More disturbingly, he stated, "The Czech Republic doesn't set the bar of what is ethical for everyone else in the region."

On several occasions, Dr. Mazur told me how deeply frustrated he was with this dominant venue-shopping mentality. Among his prospective clients, he encountered it often. For him, there was only one standard for ethics, as embodied in the Good Clinical Practice guideline. But he had clients, "especially Japanese, maybe Americans, who think you can do something in Central-Eastern Europe that is forbidden in other countries." In one case, he explained how a prospective client wanted his company's assistance in recruiting patients with moderate asthma. "The client demanded that asthma patients could be treated, but *not* with cortical steroids!" Those who are afflicted with moderate levels of asthma commonly use cortical steroids. They are available in Poland as a standard first-line treatment: "I told the client, 'Cortical steroids *must* be included in your research protocol. Patients *must* be allowed cortical steroids up to a certain dosage, because it is against treatment guidelines for asthma to withhold them.' I said to them, 'You can do whatever you want, but what you are doing is against ethical guidelines.' You won't believe how the client responded. He said, 'Okay, if we can't do this here, then why are you promoting Central-Eastern Europe?"

Insurance and Legal Protection

Two trends mark the operations of clinical research: industrialization and internationalization. In the United States and Western Europe, contract research organizations have established working partnerships with academic and medical institutions and have industrialized research. CROs have also internationalized in search of investigators and research subjects in middle- and low-income countries. The use of CROs has resulted in more competition in the clinical research market. As economist Joe Harrington put it, "An economist's natural inclination is to think that more competition is good, as it induces greater efficiency."[42] Yet my Polish and Brazilian interlocutors have made it clear that competition in this industry is intimately tied to the management of slack and to access to environments that can help compensate (with their specific resources and malfunctions) for that slack. The efficiency generated here is short-term and has its own hidden costs.[43]

Several professionals I spoke to mentioned that drug companies invest variably in quality. As I have been showing in this chapter, companies leave it up to their contractors to evaluate drug study protocols for their safety and to assess their own ability to execute the studies (their potential risks and liability) and to produce the needed evidence. For CROs, quality lies in the appropriateness of the subject pool and the expertise of investigators and study staff at the research site. There is no focus here on ethics per se. Such quality, however, is not easily observed. Subject inclusion criteria are constantly customized ("we need asthma patients who aren't taking steroids," or "we want diabetic patients with high blood-sugar levels"), as are the technical procedures to deliver results. The competitive structure of this offshoring and subcontracting affords wide latitude for problematic choices and behavior. But something else is equally important: the encroachment of this private enterprise into state regulatory and public health institutions. The efficiency and life span of clinical trials environments depend on degrees of state regulation and the extent to which health inequalities are politicized (or not).

It takes significant amounts of personnel investment and financial and political work to make offshored experimental environments work. It also takes a new mentality to assume that it is legitimate to implement protocols that violate one's own safety and ethical standards, but that might satisfy the standards of local experts and patients who "willingly" enroll in the studies. Informed by ethical variability, international and local players are unevenly situated at the contractual negotiating table. The bargaining power of locals is by and large subsumed under the desired knowledge, technologies, and monies flowing in. Patients' safety and value remain underhypothesized as clinical trials operate as social goods. As a U.S. lawyer working for a small pharmaceutical company told me in 2006, "Unfortunately, it takes an injury in clinical trials to figure out who is going to be responsible."

As Martin's temporal structure (of opportunism, peaking, and exhaustion) suggests, state regulatory mechanisms materialize fairly late in the life cycle of offshored clinical research. The Polish industry experts I spoke to characterized this third moment as riddled with "bureaucratic formalism" that would make trials too expensive and burdensome to run. They were anxiously trying to avert their industry's demise. I was interested in these debates over the adequate level of state involvement in regulation. At the same time, I wondered about the state's actual role in ensuring the protection of experimental subjects.

Officers in Poland's drug regulatory agency gave me insights into the kinds of challenges they face. These officers were either part of the country's Good Clinical Practice inspection team, created in the wake of Poland's acceptance of the EU Clinical Trial Directive, or were involved in the approval and monitoring of trials in their country. With their separate stamps of approval, Polish data can then become part of drug applications submitted to the European Agency for the Evaluation of Medicinal Products (EMEA) and the FDA.

"What are some of the problem areas that you feel particularly good about having solved?" I asked them. "The garbage trials," one officer was quick to respond, noting that her team had promoted stricter control over pediatric research, as well as other types of research that did not serve national interests. Of the four hundred new trials registered in 2004, ten were rejected, they said, for these reasons: "no insurance documents," "poor randomization ratio" (fewer patients were randomized to an expensive treatment and more to a placebo), and the case of a sponsor who "wanted to conduct a Phase 3 study without showing Phase 2 documentation." One officer conceded that his office had no precise record of how many patients were enrolled (the lack of this type of knowledge is not unique to Poland). "No one knows," he continued. "Patients can be enrolled two or three times, but we don't know for sure." The officers said they needed "sponsor-site agreement documentation," in accord with the EU directive, "so that we know who is assuming responsibility for the trial—not a virtual person." They expressed particular concern with "how *real* the patients are." Investigators are paid on a per-patient basis, and officers' task was to make sure patients and data were not being fabricated. "There are not enough checks to prevent this from happening."

My second set of questions focused on risks. "As regulators," I asked, "what is the worst kind of risk that you are trying to prevent?" They did not hesitate and answered in almost complete unison: "That a person is on a trial but does not know it." Informed consent and keeping research formally ethical (hence traceable) was their concern. The other side of this concern is the reality of trials' "becoming a normal part of health care," in Martin's words. This state of experiment-as-health care, as we will see below, constitutes an unsettled legal frontier.

As I engaged these professionals, I sensed between the lines of their speech a struggle over what kind of "face" to give to clinical research regulation in Poland. Among the industry workers, one officer, Karolina, was referred to as a potential ally of sorts. Dr. Mazur, for example, spoke about personally working with Karolina to catch instances of investigator noncompliance or misbehavior. The emphasis on maximizing patient safety and data production quality was important for Dr. Mazur, as this was Poland's differentiating brand. In his words, "Study monitors control whether investigators are doing things properly or not. Of course you cannot interfere in how investigators treat their patients. But you can report their activity somehow. If there is a risk of an investigator becoming too motivated to keep a patient on a trial, even though a drug or a placebo may be harming him, I can inform the GCP inspector, who, in turn, can have the data excluded from registration." This action can be extremely costly for pharmaceutical firms since it can raise doubts about the validity of an entire trial.

On the other hand, some research professionals blamed Polish regulators for eroding the market's confidence in the country. I heard statements such as "The bureaucrats are too slow in approving clinical trials applications" and they "require too many notarized signatures." One local executive of a multinational pharmaceutical company claimed that of late, the national drug regulatory agency was resisting taking part in establishing regional IRBs and training IRB members. "They are too worried about looking like fronts for the industry," he said. This professional told me about a recent multinational oncology trial with research sites in Western Europe and Poland. Midway through the trial, the drug company asked Polish regulators for permission to raise the number of Polish patients involved in the study, from fifty to one hundred. Regulators denied the request. He attributed this regulatory action to "some clerical notion of proportionality." Dr. Mazur concurred that the denial was off base, "since there is nothing in the EU Clinical Trial Directive concerning limits of patients per country."

One could read this event as an attempt by Polish regulators to trumpet themselves as defenders of public safety, an act that begs the question of what the role of public institutions is in "pharma-emerging" countries.[44] Clinical research attracts investments but also gives regulators in these countries the chance for their governments to exercise sovereignty as they see fit and to jockey for more say in the types of trials that are proposed. As trial environments solidify, so does this tension between public and private interests—a tension that does not necessarily stall trials but, rather, leads to continuous renegotiations over the application of law, norms, investments, and operations. Liability is also at stake. Doubling the number of Polish patients on the trial meant "doubling the risk for the government," as one regulator was quick to point out. "Who is responsible for treatment expenses that are beyond the care linked to the trial? The Polish state? The sponsor? The insurance company? We know that in the end, the Polish health-care budget will be responsible."

Clinical trial insurance requirements vary by country, and some countries eager to attract research investments agree to absorb some of the costs of medical care (linked to trial-related adverse events, for example) in their public health-care system. Insurance provides civil liability protection to a company in case of injury claims, and investigators are generally covered unless their actions deviate from protocol requirements. The most common form of insurance policy is written on a "claims made" basis, placing the claims-making burden on the injured subject. Even with insurance policies, responsibility for adverse events remains fairly circumscribed from a legal point of view; and patients are often alone in taking on the burden of proving damages, which can be a very difficult thing to do.

Insurance, I learned, is considered a costly add-on for sponsoring companies. At a 2004 global clinical research conference, I listened in an open session as the director of a small U.S. CRO (focused on dermatological studies in Latin America) lectured a representative from the Brazilian National Health Surveillance Agency (ANVISA) on how important it was "to avoid the insurance path." This representative supported legislation that would require CROs to register with ANVISA and to purchase local insurance for trials. "We want to know that if patients get injured there will be money there to take care of them," he told me in a discussion later that day: "Too often pharmaceutical companies work through third parties. A CRO comes in, runs a trial, and let's say there is an adverse event, like someone needing surgery. Generally, the CRO is not held liable, even though the pharmaceutical company guarantees liability coverage."

This Brazilian officer emphasized that beyond standard models of compliance, trial contracts need regulatory oversight, and state legislation is needed to build patient protection into those contracts. "Patients sign consent forms, but protection is a fiction. They are not insured." He is trying to create a legal environment to counter what seems to be the norm in offshored experimental environments: that it takes injury, scandal, or sustained patient advocacy to hold trial sponsors accountable, and to institute fairer terms than are assumed in the contract of the standard "social good" kind of trial. Reversing this norm takes a great deal of political effort and the design of alternative practices of research (see chapter 4).

I was referred to a Warsaw-based lawyer, whom I will call Piotr, who represents pharmaceutical companies in clinical trials litigation. Piotr's mission in the courts, as I would learn, was to minimize the link between civil liability and clinical trials and to convince judges that clinical trials participation was a form of medical treatment. Young and well-dressed, this ambitious-sounding lawyer told me that medical laws regulating clinical trials have been enforced since 2002 and that previously there had been "almost no cases" of trial subject litigation. "Patients are becoming much more aggressive in their legal strategies," Piotr told me. He blamed negative media portrayals and the encroachment of American litigation culture. "If they do not secure damages from a sponsor's insurance, they go to court." Piotr told me he has seen three cases of patient litigation since 2003. "Is that a lot or a little?" I asked him. He thought that was a lot.

But he believed that litigants' chances of winning in court were slim. "The tradition of medical malpractice law in Eastern Europe is weak," Piotr pointed out. "Patients will experience great difficulty in making claims against sponsors for damages that they allege are trial related." He was in the midst of defending one drug company, attempting to frame the case of an adverse event (a death) that occurred during a trial as being related to "physician abuse, a protocol violation." Piotr and his peers work to maintain a favorable legal environment for the trial enterprise. The judicial system is a key battlefield because, as he noted, "court decisions can go either way," and this leaves room for lawyers to create industry-favoring precedents, like that of physician abuse.

Piotr told me he had recently won a court battle involving a trial in which a new treatment was compared to a standard treatment. A patient on the standard arm of the trial alleged damages. "But in this case, the standard treatment was registered in Poland. I argued that product liability regulation should rule, not clinical trials regulation. The lower court accepted this reasoning." In other words, only the subjects treated in a nonstandard way had a right to litigate. The rest of the trial subjects were just consumers, "as if they were not taking part in a clinical trial at all." This is the legal underside of normalizing the clinical trial as a medical alternative within the public health-care system. Piotr was optimistic that the Polish Supreme Court would "react positively" to his arguments. "These kinds of claims are new," he said. "There is no final decision yet. The rules are not clear. There will be more judicial rulings. All I can do is formulate general principles, but I cannot formulate specifics, that is, the decisions of the court. But at this point, no one can say what kinds of rights patients have and what kinds of rights patients don't have."

My trip to Poland was nearly over, but the industry professionals I had engaged would continue to be preoccupied with the expiration date of the Polish clinical trials environment. These individuals would persist in promoting trials, recruiting experts, leveraging large subject cohorts, tinkering with protocols, trying to influence the regulatory environment. As they continued to actively shape the public's understandings of clinical trials—their benefit to patients and to public health writ large—concerns over what medical value clinical trials participation actually provided were beginning to emerge and to garner media attention. In probing the characteristics of the research environment, I have shown some of the challenges in tracking clinical trials, maintaining scientific integrity, and minimizing research-related harms. The meaning of vulnerability lies not only in a priori categories of vulnerable persons or populations, but also in everyday ethical and legal decisions that can put power out of the reach of patients and leave them exposed to multiple risks. The political subjectivities and jurisprudence that form in the wake of the globalized trial have to be tracked. They speak to the conundrums that people are left with in the aftermath of trials, and to how accountability can be brought to bear on this hypermobile off-shored enterprise.

CHAPTER FOUR

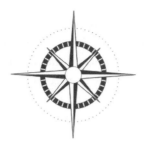

PHARMACEUTICALS AND THE
RIGHT TO HEALTH

Reclaiming Patients and the Evidence Base of Drugs

So far, I have been chronicling the offshoring of clinical trials and inquiring into the new experimental environments that are emerging internationally. The pharmaceutical industry has disaggregated core processes of drug development (such as clinical research) and rebuilt them in new locations, where it obtains access to skilled professionals and lower-cost infrastructures. Sitting in an elegant Warsaw office in 2005, a medical director of a multinational drug firm stressed the nonlocal character of clinical research: "We get the protocols from the research and development department in U.S. headquarters. We have no locally designed study." This American-trained Polish physician managed teams of young researchers and coordinated clinical trials in different therapeutic areas in the region. He worked directly with local investigators or with locally based contract research organizations when necessary, and he explained how productive Central-Eastern Europe is in terms of patient data (second only to the United States). This professional explained that companies weigh each world region's productivity in terms of output of clinical research units (CRUs), a measure of the labor-intensiveness involved in the monitoring of a single trial subject. "In our formula, we multiply the value of the patient by his or her complexity. So one patient in an oncology study is like two patients in a respiratory or simple hypertension study. We are doing a lot of CRUs in Poland. We are still trailing behind the U.S. in terms of CRUs, but we are ahead of Latin America by five years."

Similar stories of productivity, competitiveness, and optimism echo around the globe. In 2004, a director of clinical research for a large drug firm located in Rio de Janeiro boasted that Brazil's clinical trials market is "one of the fastest growing in the world." He estimated that about 95 percent of his company's work involved multicentered trials in second and third phases. "For instance, at the moment I have around twenty-five different protocols. These protocols can involve research subjects from up to seventy countries. I am working with only one locally designed protocol." He emphasized the benefits of this enterprise: "Yes, a lot of data are transferred out of the country, yet a lot of clinical investment comes back in."

This professional was confident about the quality of the Brazilian clinical research data. "International guidelines are in place locally." Both he and his Polish counterpart defended the value structure of transnational drug development—ensured by patent-related agreements, ethical guidelines, and regulatory standards governing trial conduct and guaranteeing the easy transferability of data.[1] They affirmed the efficacy and transparency of a global clinical trials system and the ability of local partners to play by its rules. The same system that holds investigators tethered to a procedural form of ethics—"No one pays better attention to the ethical guidelines than us," in the words of the Brazilian expert—also works to redefine patient data as intellectual property and to limit the terms of its use. Lost in all the industry success stories are simple questions: How do data figure back into local health systems, if at all? What are the implications of the short- and long-term withholding of patient data? Equally critical, what is the actual value of drugs, and what value do patients impart to this enterprise?

Some physicians who occasionally run industry-sponsored trials question the value that research brings to public health. As Dr. Raul Amos, a Brazilian physician, remarked, "I give the patient the meds and measure the endpoints. Just measure and send the data off electronically. By the end of the trial we have sent a lot of raw data to the company." From his perspective, conformity and intellectual passivity on the part of local investigators underpin the value structure so heavily prized by the purveyors of the globalized trial. As I learned in Poland, some physicians who were considered to be too sympathetic toward patients and public health needs could not be trusted to carry out industry-sponsored research. They were branded as potential "protocol violators" who had a tendency to overenroll patients for medical care purposes. Arguably, there and elsewhere, physician-investigators are valued to the extent that they can turn patients into health-care consumers, embedding them in global experimental networks, all the while distancing themselves from the public health implications of their work. As industry-sponsored research merges seamlessly with the habits and routines of health care, Dr. Amos remarked, "All there is left for me to do is to follow the rules and recommendations. They have bought almost everyone."

Yet there are alternatives to this dire image of the medical homo economicus. In this chapter, I explore how a team of academic researchers at a southern Brazilian university hospital (hereafter, the hospital) is trying to reverse the troubling forms of business control that have evolved over medical science and care on the ground. They are concerned not only with the loss of professional autonomy, but with the public health impact of valuing patient data solely in industrial terms. How is local health care—public and individual—compromised? They are also concerned with the aftermath of clinical trials and ensuring future treatments for patients in trials. In the words of one team member who conducts studies on genetic therapies that can cost hundreds of thousands of dollars per patient annually: "We have to deal with the problems that begin when the study ends, particularly the continuity of treatment, the right dosages, and the quality of care as patients return to their hometowns."

Once clinical trial data have been sent off to corporate headquarters, new medical fields emerge locally. Issues such as continuity of treatment and ongoing control of data by sponsors pose specific medical challenges. Patients require treatments that are now on the market and out of their reach, and trial sponsors still try to maintain control over patient data in the drug-marketing phase. There are also escalating demands imposed by patients and marketers on doctors to prescribe, and on the state to provide, new high-cost medicines, some of whose clinical benefits are not unequivocally established. What is the adequate response to citizens' demands for these pharmaceuticals?

These issues are salient in the United States, where health care is fragmented and privatized. In what follows, I trace some of the public and private tensions of health-care delivery in Brazil. I explore how local doctors, families, and patients become agentive forces in a rapidly growing drug market, where public health resources remain scarce. We will observe the concrete and contentious ways in which a group of academic scientists subjects a micro-medical economy to an adjudicating clinical science. In doing so, they reclaim patients (and patient data) and embed them in new health-care networks, regional and national, rather than in global medical markets. These scientists are also taking up a key global health challenge: health technology assessment or "how to guarantee access to medicines without resorting to treatment triage or severely crippling already limited public health budgets," as Dr. Paulo Picon, who has spearheaded these efforts, told me at our first meeting in 2003. Health technology assessment is an international movement that strives for evidence-based decision making in health-care policies and practices. "It is not a matter of rejecting new technologies. If the drugs do good, we will be happy to use them. And we are using them as much as we can. But we have to find clear and safe treatment criteria and to monitor patients in the long run."

This search for clear and safe treatment criteria is controversial, but it can lead to new domestic research capacities that can potentially revitalize the role of academic medicine in global health. What are the ethics and politics of this kind of experimentality? What sorts of complicities and compromises are involved? How can this alternative technological capacity inform domestic health policy?

"Pharmaceuticals are the new gold"

"The entire society is being recruited by the pharmaceutical industry," Dr. Picon told me during an August 2004 conversation in his hospital office. Opened in 1971, the hospital is a center of excellence in health care, teaching, and research and is considered one of the ten best public hospitals in Brazil, boasting more than sixty medical specialties. More than three hundred professors from the Federal University of Rio Grande do Sul (UFRGS) work there and train an average of three hundred medical residents.

Dr. Picon received his medical training at the Federal University and earned a Ph.D. in cardiology in a joint program with a prestigious American medical school. He has trained scores of medical students in clinical pharmacology and evidenced-based medicine, understood as the "conscientious, explicit, and judicious use of current best evidence" in clinical decision making.[2] His students, who have gone on to become doctoral candidates, residents, doctors, and pharmacists, form the core of his health technology assessment group.[3] Dr. Picon also serves in various public positions. He is an adviser to the country's Ministry of Health and the Brazilian National Health Surveillance Agency (ANVISA), as well as a health authority in the state of Rio Grande do Sul. The fifty-year-old scientist had just been named director of the hospital's Clinical Research Unit. Opened in 2003, the unit is one of eight national centers devoted to bioequivalence studies of generic drugs.

At the time of our meeting, Dr. Picon was leading a national scientific task force focusing on public access to high-cost medicines. In Brazil these medicines are also known as exceptional medicines (*medicamentos excepcionais*). The Ministry of Health purchases and distributes them in an exceptional way, that is, with monies that are not part of the universal health-care system or national disease programs. Demand for exceptional medicines is growing; many patient groups that already receive exceptional medicines want their treatment programs to become part of a national disease program. AIDS and tuberculosis treatments constitute such national programs and are based on centralized purchasing. Such purchasing, patient groups argue, guarantees reliable access and resolves irregularities of regional and municipal pharmaceutical assistance programs.[4] Aspects of this access system need reassessment as, according to Dr. Picon, "some of these drugs are aggressively marketed, but many of them have an incomplete evidence base." Drug value is as much a topic of scientific debate as it is a contested political and economic matter. What I heard Dr. Picon and colleagues stating repeatedly is that when the government is the primary buyer, the value of drugs must be thoroughly scrutinized. He referred to drug-marketing practices as predatory, even toxic: "They make the poison, and we have to make the counterpoison."

Dr. Picon travels and lectures widely. At the beginning of his PowerPoint presentations he declares, "No conflicts of interest. No financial relationship to any multinational pharmaceutical or medical device company." He recalled the day a drug company representative interrupted him during rounds in the hospital's emergency room. The representative wanted to meet with him to discuss a drug that was under Brazilian regulatory review. "The guy just assumed that I was available for him. It was totally invasive. If you keep opening the door, you lose control over your medical practice and you never get it back."

Over the past decade, this physician-scientist has observed with alarm how the industry has influenced the course of academic medicine and public health in Brazil. "They know all the strategies and use knowledge with extreme efficiency. When you create a rule, they know how to bypass it." Companies sponsor trips, hand out gifts, finance conferences. "Some physicians prescribe the medication that the company wants him to prescribe, and the patient never questions the physician," Dr. Picon added. There has been a steep rise in lawsuits brought by citizens against the state to obligate the state to provide high-cost drugs. The median income of the wealthiest 10 percent of the population is almost thirty times greater than that of the poorest 40 percent.[5] Access to medicines as a human right is a crucial remedy for these grossly disparate income levels. But patients "from all social classes" are demanding such drugs from state and municipal health secretariats. Private lawyers and public prosecutors working for the Public Ministry (a body of magistrates who can bring actions against federal, state, or municipal governments in defense of citizens' rights) are being called to represent patients, and, in the end, local judges frequently decide in favor of providing treatments. "What isn't in the file is the evidence to back up the claim that the drug works or the commercial interests behind the claim," Dr. Picon said.[6]

Brazil is the second largest pharmaceutical market in Latin America, after Mexico. With a population of roughly 190 million people, the country moved from a dictatorship to democratic government in the mid-1980s. Since then, it has recast its economy according to new global trade rules largely under the government of Fernando Henrique Cardoso (1995–2002). State industries were rapidly privatized, social spending was reduced, and services were decentralized. In 1996, the country changed its patent legislation and complied with the TRIPS (trade-related aspects of intellectual property rights) Agreement. TRIPS ushered in a new ecology of international trade regulation. It introduced standards for the legal protection and enforcement of intellectual property, including pharmaceutical product patents, and guaranteed exclusive marketing rights. With trade-friendly intellectual property legislation, Brazil attracted new pharmaceutical investments and dramatically increased imports of medicines. By 2000, however, the initial strong growth in pharmaceutical commerce had slowed somewhat. Investors became cautious when the government threatened to break patents on AIDS drugs and introduced a program for generic drugs. The fact is that pharmaceuticals, be they brand-name or generics, have penetrated the fabric of communities everywhere, while a large number of Brazilians still die of infectious rather than chronic diseases. Sales of antidepressants, lifestyle drugs, and blockbuster drugs have soared. A striking paradox is now routinized: you might be out of work or hungry but you could still claim your free antianxiety pill, for example, at a local health post.[7]

President Luis Inacio Lula da Silva of the Worker's Party (Partido dos Trabalhadores, PT), now in his second term, has more or less adhered to the economic orthodoxies of his predecessor by supporting a floating exchange rate and instituting inflationary targets and strict fiscal policies. Brazil is struggling to sustain its economic growth and highly unequal income distribution remains an urgent problem. The social field is marked by economic insecurity, violence, and a fierce battle over scarce state resources. For many, citizenship has been equated with accessing income supplements and medical treatments. Anthropologist João Biehl refers to this process as the "pharmaceuticalization" of health-care delivery (2006, 2007).[8]

Dr. Andry Costa, a cardiologist who is part of Dr. Picon's technology assessment task force, does not blame patients alone for the voracious pharmaceutical demand. He attributes it to an unholy mixture of aggressive marketing, a lack of stricter state regulation, and a general bias among patients for brand-name medicines. He insists on the crucial role of academic medicine in creating mechanisms to ensure the right administration of new therapies. He explained, "Specialists prescribe the newer drugs, while general physicians can easily treat many problems with one or two older drugs." Patients are inundated with me-too drugs. "Those who come to see me with heart problems often have two or three prescriptions for the same drug, but under different brand names, and with dosages that are way too high. Many don't even know what they are taking. Do I interrupt all their treatments and start from scratch? It's a real mess."

The story gets even more complicated when seen from the perspective of distressed patients and their families who know of the existence of effective and potentially lifesaving treatments but cannot access them. For too long, state-of-the-art treatments have not been commonly made available to the poorest. AIDS and medical activists have shown that it is "cost-effective" to treat the poor and that the industry can be pressured to lower drug prices.[9] Moreover, as I learned from the mother of a patient being treated for a rare disorder, treatment activism—suing the state—forces the government to make important administrative changes that can improve health-care delivery. In 1993, after much difficulty in obtaining the correct diagnosis, the Souzas, Lucia and her husband Luis, waged a desperate battle to obtain treatment for their five-year-old son Pedro, who suffered from Type 1 Gaucher disease, a condition that is treated by a drug that can cost more than $200,000 per year. The lower-middle-class family had been living in a northern state where the couple worked at a medical school.

Since he was a toddler, Pedro had suffered from anemia, and his spleen and liver were enlarged. "My husband and I didn't know that we are carriers of the gene mutation. It was destiny. We met, fell in love, and had a child." Lucia recalled their medical odyssey: "First the pediatrician, and then, from specialist to specialist, it took us more than two years to find out what Pedro had. We realized that most doctors did not know about genetic diseases, and when they said they knew, they also said that there was no treatment. Finally, a geneticist told us that it might be Gaucher disease and that we might get a dose of an enzymatic treatment from a hospital in São Paulo or Porto Alegre."

Gaucher is a rare inherited disorder in which an enzyme deficiency results in gradual blood, bone, and, in some cases, nervous impairment. A first version of enzyme replacement therapy needed to treat Gaucher had been approved by the FDA and marketed in the United States. "Since we were from the state of Rio Grande do Sul and had family here, I got a leave from my job and we came to the hospital to investigate. It took one visit, one blood sample, and we finally had the right diagnosis." The parents went to the state's health secretariat and requested the therapy. "A few months passed and state health officials did not give us any assurance that the treatment would be available. We had heard of a rich family in Rio de Janeiro who bought the drug directly from the manufacturer. We were one of the first families here to file a lawsuit, and we won. In 1994, the judge granted us the right to treatment."

With a court injunction in hand, the couple went back to the state health officials, obtaining a promise that tens of thousand of dollars would be wired to them so that they could buy the drug directly from the manufacturer. "My husband still has the first bottle. It was like winning the lottery." Soon, many other families would follow in their footsteps, and well-organized and vocal Gaucher families throughout the country would keep struggling for reliable treatment access. In 1995, they succeeded in having Gaucher listed as a national disease program.[10] In 1997, the manufacturer opened a Brazilian office to coordinate its market, research, and public outreach activities in the country.

Health Technology Assessment in Brazil

Pharmaceutical assistance is an integral part of Brazil's universal healthcare policy. The country's progressive constitution of 1988 guaranteed its citizens universal access to health as a basic right. "Health is the right of all and the duty of the state. It is guaranteed by social and economic policies that reduce the risk of disease and other adversities and by universal and equal access to actions and services."[11] Through the national health system (Sistema Único de Saúde, or SUS), health coverage was ostensibly extended to all citizens, including those covered outside the system.[12] While the federal government retained a role in financing public health, states and municipalities began administering federal funds. They also had to cofinance the development of new health infrastructures and facilities.

Until 1992, the federal government was responsible for the acquisition and distribution of exceptional medicines—primarily, at the time, cyclosporine for transplant patients and erythropoietin for patients with anemia and chronic renal disease. That year, the Health Ministry placed the program for exceptional medicines under the control of state health secretariats—but without a well-defined cofinancing mechanism. In 1996, new criteria for making the program work were defined, and the list of exceptional medicines expanded to include 32 drugs. By 2002, the program financed the purchase and distribution of 104 drugs at a cost of roughly $250 million for some 130,000 patients.

Mounting demands for high-cost treatment for diseases ranging from hepatitis C to Alzheimer's, Parkinson's, and severe asthma to genetic disorders, schizophrenia, rheumatoid arthritis, and bipolar disorder reflect public health transitions in poor and middle-income countries. As mortality rates from infectious diseases drop, chronic diseases like heart disease and stroke become greater health problems. Changing patterns of mortality and disease occur in tandem with the introduction of new medical technologies, social mobilization (in the case of Brazil), and marketing pressures. While state-purchased exceptional medicines make up a fast-growing and formidable market in Brazil, citizens still find that drugs from the country's list of essential medicines are unavailable in local pharmacies.

Drug firms, capitalizing on the idea of citizen empowerment, have used the progressive human rights instrument as a way of disseminating their products. The question of access or, rather, of the sustainability of established national treatment programs (for AIDS, for example) bears directly on the issue of evidence-based decision making in health care. The availability of and access to high-cost drugs has prompted the government to rethink its drug-purchasing policies and rationalize their use. In 2000, then health minister José Serra invited Dr. Picon to lead an effort to establish a mechanism "to guarantee safe and efficacious prescription" of exceptional medicines—which ultimately led to the 2002 publication of the *Clinical Protocols and Therapeutic Guidelines: Exceptional Medicines* (*Protocolos Clínicos e Diretrizes Terapêuticas: Medicamentos Excepcionais,* hereafter *Protocolos*). In Dr. Picon's words, "The Health Ministry wanted us to make sense of all this. Up until then, the ministry was just a good payer. It just paid for these medicines. It never measured health outcomes and bought drugs of unproven value for our people. It never published anything. There were no scientific criteria or tools in place to evaluate high-cost drugs and to integrate them in the universal health-care system. It was all a matter of how much pressure society and drug company reps put on the health ministry and what drugs' package inserts said in terms of their use."

Minister Serra had played a critical role in sustaining the Brazilian AIDS treatment rollout. By reverse engineering antiretroviral drugs and promoting the production of generics in public and private laboratories, the Health Ministry created mechanisms for drug price differentiation. Such differentiation kept the rollout in place, which in turn led to significant drops in hospitalization rates and AIDS mortality.[13] But for all the good it had done, I frequently heard from health professionals that the AIDS policy had also opened the floodgates for high-cost drugs. In 2002, the Ministry of Health spent about $1 billion on drugs. In 2005, this expenditure had reached close to $2 billion. If in 2002, pharmaceutical assistance took up 5.8 percent of the country's health budget, in 2005, it took up 8.5 percent (Messeder 2005). Arguably, access to all kinds of medicines, whether they are on the country's essential drug list, part of specialized programs, or even in experimental stages and not yet approved for marketing, have come to stand in for the right to health. "We are all being used to test, approve, or market drugs that have an unproven value for our people," the cardiologist Dr. Costa stated.

Just as the country had created a successful price-negotiation strategy to secure AIDS therapies, now it needed institutional mechanisms to address and reverse the new problems linked to the influx of high-cost medicines and pharmaceuticalization. Minister Serra, for example, waged a fierce battle with one multinational drug firm over its alleged "abusive" pricing practices. The company, Serra charged, was taking advantage of Brazil's constitutional right to universal health care and manipulating its court system. For example, it was mobilizing patient groups to demand its twice-as-expensive drug over the available generic, used to prevent organ rejection in kidney, liver, and heart transplant patients (Ramos 2005).

The universalizing of high-cost drugs is a human rights triumph, but access to essential medicines remains uncertain. While the federal allocation for essential medicines for the general population remained around $75 million per year between 2002 and 2005, the joint budget for AIDS therapies and exceptional medicines that supports the treatment of a few hundred thousand people, for example, climbed to well over $1 billion in the same period (Messeder 2005). Other high-cost drugs came on the scene in the wake of Brazil's AIDS drugs–purchasing policies, and the *Protocolos* were to provide guidelines aimed at ensuring widespread consistency in their administration and optimally effective uses.

Clinical practice guidelines abound in medicine. They are products of expert assessments and accumulated evidence, but, as Timmermans and Berg write, they also "indicate the mixed feelings professionals have toward the standardization of their work processes. . . . Professions express a love-hate relationship toward standards in general, and clinical practice guidelines in particular" (2003:84). Yet it would be a mistake to frame the efforts of the Brazilian guidelines as mere technocratic exercises in drug cost containment or standardization. The *Protocolos* speak to a large-scale public health experiment that comes with drugs and their unmonitored and haphazard use. They address a nonstandard patient in need of personalized treatment based on longitudinal observation. The focus here is on clinical specificities and on how to improve clinical outcomes with the drugs that are already available. This particularized approach is "patient- and not specialist-centered," Dr. Picon told me. "Brazilian real-life patients are much sicker than the ideal patients in clinical trials. The unrealistic scenarios of randomized controlled trials are prone to produce biased data." Through the consideration of the "real-life patient," issues of appropriate dosage or whether treatments and retreatments are actually suitable or dangerous can be investigated and resolved.

Dr. Picon proudly showed me the thick *Protocolos* manual, filled with carefully presented data and easy-to-read flowcharts. The manual contains thirty-one clinical protocols and therapeutic guidelines for the prescription of exceptional medicines that have passed through a public consultation.[14] The *Protocolos* review the clinical situation to be treated and disease classification and present diagnostic criteria as well as criteria for treatment inclusion and exclusion. Special cases whose risks and benefits must be assessed by physicians are also listed. There is an extensive presentation of treatment options and their bases (description of medicines and their administration, as well as length of treatment and potential benefits). They conclude with a description of monitoring strategies and lists of possible side effects and counterindications for various medicines. Patients and doctors sign informed consent forms, thus agreeing to this local treatment order. Dr. Picon received a National Order of Merit for this particular effort, and he was eager to have the *Protocolos* implemented around the country. He and his team, however, faced strong resistance from medical opinion makers and envisioned an uphill battle against corporate and specialized medical interests.

The Judicialization of Health

During our first collective meeting in June 2003, the *Protocolos* task force spoke at length about the inequities of the global pharmaceutical reality that the country was part of. Residents talked about high-cost "orphan drugs"—of the kind the Souzas fought to get for their son and for which Brazil was becoming a major market. These markets, they said, were also related to regulatory mandates and incentives in the North. The 1983 U.S. Orphan Drug Act provides incentives for the development of drugs to treat rare diseases affecting "less than 200,000 persons in the U.S." or "more than 200,000 persons in the U.S. but for which there is no reasonable expectation that the cost of developing and making available in the U.S. a drug for such disease or condition will be recovered from sales in the U.S. of such drug."[15] These incentives include tax credits for clinical research and seven years of market exclusivity for an FDA-approved drug. They specifically talked about a drug used to treat acute myeloid leukemia. The FDA granted approval for imatinib (known as Gleevec in the United States) in May 2001 in what was one of the fastest review periods of any cancer drug.[16]

"This is a good drug," said Dr. Picon. "There is no doubt that it works. The problem is its price and the inability of the scientific community to influence price control." Initially the average cost of the drug in the United States and worldwide was estimated to be $2,500 per month, depending on the dosage. In 2004, the average cost was closer to $3,500 per month, and sales reached $1.57 billion (Ramos 2004). Sales reached more than $2 billion in 2006 and are expected to reach $2.73 billion in 2008.[17] Under normal conditions, drug costs should drop. But because of lack of competition the prices of orphan drugs can remain inordinately high. In the United States, poorer patients took advantage of the manufacturer's patient assistance programs.

In Brazil, people enrolled in trials to access this treatment. According to Dr. Picon, "The manufacturer sought approval from ANVISA. And in order to be approved, it needed to carry out studies in the country. If it were to be approved here, it would be approved elsewhere in South America." He attended a regional experts meeting at which imatinib was debated among medical experts. "I made the case that at least trial patients should benefit from lifelong treatment, paid for by the company." Dr. Picon was dismayed to learn that posttrial treatment would be the government's responsibility. Capitalizing on citizen empowerment, the company argued that "patients needed to exercise their right to health and pressure the government to purchase the drug." The issue of price was elided.

Litigation has become a common pathway for patients to access high-cost drugs that are not yet covered by pharmaceutical assistance programs, as well as drugs that are included in national programs but that are not locally available. The number of legal suits filed by patients against municipal and state health departments has skyrocketed throughout Brazil in the last decade. While 1,126 suits were brought against the state of Rio Grande do Sul in 2002, in 2005 this number rose to 4,855 (Picon 2006). In 2001, the municipal health secretary of Goiânia, the capital of the central-western state of Goias, spent on average 10,000 dollars per month to fulfill court injunctions for the dispensation of exceptional medicines. In 2006, this expense was close to 50,000 dollars per month (half the resources allocated for the purchase of essential medicines).[18]

Dr. Guilherme Sander, a gastroenterologist and one of Picon's collaborators, spoke bitterly against this now-entrenched litigation culture. Desperate patients are motivated by inadequate medical care, he said, or "have been convinced by advertising of the effectiveness of experimental treatments." Dr. Sander described lawyers standing outside hospitals and offering to litigate rights to health for patients and families; he was critical about the "blind introduction" of therapeutic innovations, particularly in university hospitals. Dr. Sander mentioned pegylated interferon to treat hepatitis C as an example of how expensive medicines with marginal improvement are taken up in the public health system. "After one molecular change," he said, "the price of the treatment went from $1,000 to $18,000. Today, we practically have no more prescriptions for standard interferon." There are about five thousand known hepatitis C patients in the country, and "demands for second and even third treatments are mushrooming. The problem is that some patients have multiple diseases. Because of a lawsuit we had to treat a cardiac transplant patient with hepatitis C with pegylated interferon, but this is contraindicated. But if the judge says you have to treat, you can't say no." Dr. Andry Costa, who was participating in the conversation, added that the patient's legal claim to a treatment is always framed in terms of life or death: "No judge wants to be held responsible for a patient's death, not the doctor, not the judge." In contexts of dire need and scarcity, this health-seeking strategy has also become a tool for everyday needs, with citizens demanding "everything from special milk to geriatric diapers."[19]

Ana Márcia Messeder and colleagues profiled this judicial phenomenon in the state of Rio de Janeiro (2005). The authors identified a total of 2,733 legal suits filed between January 1991 and December 2002 and analyzed a representative sample of 389 of them (14 percent of the total). They found that the majority of cases were initiated by public defenders or pro bono lawyers from NGOs or universities and that only 16 percent of the legal suits came from patients being treated outside of the national health system. By the end of the study, more than 80 percent of the cases had not been adjudicated. AIDS patients were the primary litigants until the late 1990s, when the universal distribution of antiretroviral drugs was regularized. A growing demand for exceptional medicines ensued: "Users of these drugs are exerting greater organizational and lobbying skills to secure their rights" (ibid.:532).

In the last years of the study, however, Messeder et al. identified a growing demand for chronic disorder treatments that had already been listed as essential medicines in the universal health-care system. This newer phenomenon might indicate the failure of municipal administrations (the supposed providers) and state health secretariats (the supposed cofinancers) to fulfill their duties to provide essential drugs (ibid.). According to the authors, public defenders and judges lack clarity about the division of pharmaceutical responsibility among various administrative levels and even show "disregard for the rational use of medicine and for possible harms that come with misprescription and misuse" (ibid.:533).

In states where municipal-level pharmaceutical programs are relatively well-functioning, most legal claims have focused on access to high-cost treatments. In Paraná, for example, the amount spent on court injunctions went from $66,000 in 2003 to almost $6 million in 2006. In 2003, the state of Minas Gerais spent $8 million on exceptional medicines. In 2004, there were 1,050 court injunctions for the state to provide medicines not covered by its pharmaceutical program. Spending jumped to $25 million—half of the total spent on pharmaceuticals in that state.[20]

The litigiousness over the right to health is woven out of many different threads, including social mobilization anchored in long histories of citizen exclusion from formal legal mechanisms, fragile health systems, industry marketing, "pharmaceuticalized" approaches to health, medically uninformed judges, and a general "judicialization" of politics (Sieder, Schjolden, and Angell 2005). Dr. Picon and his team are concerned with the lack of rigorous medical review and with public health equity as the relentless wheel of the pharmaceuticalization and judicialization of health rolls on. "Forget about the rules. Forget about treatment protocols. Forget about the rational use of medicines." If a doctor prescribes a treatment and a judge validates the claim, Dr. Picon added, "then local health authorities must provide the treatment in three days. Physicians or local health administrators who do not provide the treatment can be arrested. Judges can issue injunctions to divert social security funds to satisfy these claims. We all wonder about what will happen with basic and preventive health care and to SUS [the national health system] in the process."[21]

Alternative Treatment Guidelines

From a health management perspective, clinical research and public health practice remain by and large disconnected. As Dr. Kamran Abbasi, former deputy editor of the *British Medical Journal*, noted, "Fewer than 5 percent of studies in medical journals are both valid and relevant to clinicians or policy makers; in most journals it's less than 1 percent" (2005). When new medicines are thrown into emerging pharmaceutical markets like Brazil and Poland, this disconnect can widen and generate new sorts of public health problems. Dr. Picon, of course, is not alone in questioning the validity of randomized controlled trials as the gold standard source of evidence (Vitoria, Habicht, and Bryce 2004), let alone claims to the therapeutic significance of new treatments as far as actual patients are concerned. I had been telling him about cardiology trials in Poland when he said, "Poland is an excellent place to run cardiology trials, so of course companies are going to perform the studies there because they have a perfect technical environment there. But in real life things will work out differently. In the end, all we know is that many of the new drugs can't kill, but we don't know if they can save, let alone how cost-effective they are."

The *Protocolos* address some of the unknowns that new therapeutic entities are introducing into routine clinical care and public health. Dr. Picon's team studied industry recommendations in drug package inserts and combed through scientific literature, comparing the efficacy claims of new drugs against the known efficacy of older ones. They analyzed the design of clinical trials, looked for flaws in the data, and identified understudied aspects. As they scrutinized trial results, they also parsed out differences in the contexts of trials and showed how results (health outcomes, rates of complication, mortality rates) in one context do not necessarily hold true for another. Then they drafted guidelines reflecting the best evidence base, recommending dosage and frequency of a drug's administration according to the severity of the disease and other individual adjustments.

All of these guidelines were posted on the Ministry of Health's Web site for open public commentary and criticism. "We were looking for some medical consensus," one member explained. But that is not what happened. The guideline for rheumatoid arthritis, for example, presciently warned against the use of COX-2 inhibitors (nonsteroidal anti-inflammatory drugs used in treating arthritis, acute pain conditions, and dysmenorrhoea) because of "indications of heart attack" (Picon and Beltrame 2002:81). During the guideline's open commentary period, the team received "26.8 kilograms of letters of complaint. Lots of experts, doctors, and chairs of medical departments urged us to recommend Vioxx to all rheumatoid arthritis patients instead of the nonexpensive and safer nonselective COX-inhibitors."

One *Protocolos* contributor said that the project threatened medical autonomies. But the letters they received indicated anything but autonomy: "They followed the same template. The order of paragraphs had been changed on some of them. The only real difference was the signature." Dr. Picon has a photograph of these packages of letters (they were delivered to him piled in a wheelchair) and shows it in his lectures to illustrate conflicts of interest in medicine and the need for an objective health technology assessment program in the country.

The treatment guideline for Gaucher disease was especially contested. It provides a good example of how difficult it is to "translate evidence into practice." Gaucher disease, as briefly described earlier, is a genetic disorder in which a person lacks an enzyme called glucocerebrosidase.[22] The lack of the enzyme causes harmful substances to build up in the liver, spleen, bones, and bone marrow, preventing them from working properly. Type 1 Gaucher disease is most common, and it involves bone disease, anemia, an enlarged spleen, and thrombocytopenia. It can be treated with imiglucerase, an enzyme replacement therapy (ERT) in which a genetically engineered form of the missing enzyme is administered intravenously.[23] The first version of the treatment (alglucerase) was approved by the FDA in 1991, and the new version, imiglucerase, gained approval in 1994—both under the Orphan Drug Act. The price of imiglucerase has not significantly dropped.[24]

There is no doubt that imiglucerase can stop or undo progressive organ damage. Patients greatly benefit from this treatment and are able to live normal and relatively healthy lives. Recall Pedro, who began taking the drug at age of three and is now a thriving young man. Yet Dr. Picon and colleagues reckon with the question of drug pricing and drug dosaging. He explained that the drug was FDA approved on the basis of a small Phase 2 study, and the standard industry-prescribed dose (of 60 units per kilogram of body weight every two weeks) is based on that initial study. "A minimum effective dose was never established in a Phase 3 trial." At the industry-prescribed dose, the roughly 500 Brazilian patients in need of the drug constitute an annual market of some $100 million.

In order to construct the Gaucher treatment guideline for the public universal health-care system, team members consulted with Dr. Ernest Beutler, a professor in the Department of Molecular and Experimental Medicine at the Scripps Research Institute in California, who had previously worked at the National Institutes of Health. In 1991, Dr. Beutler published the first major study of the natural history of the disease. They also contacted Dr. Ari Zimran, a former research fellow of Dr. Beutler, and director of the Gaucher Clinic at Shaare Zedek Medical Center in Israel. With more than five hundred patients, this is the largest Gaucher clinic in the world. Dr. Beutler and Dr. Zimran reported positive clinical results with significantly lower doses than those recommended by the drug manufacturer. Dr. Beutler published an editorial in the *American Journal of Medicine* alleging "economic malpractice" in the treatment of Gaucher disease. He recounted how company representatives had tried to shift his patients to other doctors because of his low-dose prescription patterns.[25] The company, he wrote, "advocat[es] doses of their drug that are four to eight times larger than those needed to provide an optimal response" (1994:2).

Dr. Picon told me that it was difficult to find Brazilian doctors to work as consultants for this specific guideline. And "comparing our data with Beutler's and Zimran's evidence, we ended up recommending fifteen units per kilogram as the initial dose, or four times less than what was recommended in the package insert, every fifteen days." The national Gaucher treatment guideline follows the Beutler and Zimran example that a significantly lower dosage of imiglucerase is effective. The guideline also provides clinical criteria for treatment inclusion and exclusion. It recommends that patients of a Gaucher Type 2 disease and asymptomatic patients should not be put on treatment. It also recommends the creation of regional reference centers to evaluate, treat, and follow up patients. A regional database would collate patient data from various reference centers to facilitate a national Gaucher database (Picon and Beltrame 2002:218).

Dr. Picon reasoned that if these measures were to be implemented, treatment costs would dramatically drop and patients would get consistent access to this much-needed treatment. But pressure came from all sides to abandon this known alternative treatment regimen. During the open commentary period for the Gaucher treatment guideline, Dr. Picon was handed "2,500 pages of complaint from industry representatives and physicians. We also received letters from a major U.S. government medical research center criticizing the guideline." The anti-*Protocolos* campaigners deployed the language of international law and human rights. "We received a letter from a lawyer representing patients saying that he would take our team to an International Criminal Court." The threat never materialized.

What is at stake in this battle over control over a drug's evidence base and patient data? Imiglucerase was approved on the basis of a small pivotal study involving twelve patients: "the investigators wisely used a very generous dose of enzyme [60 units/kg] to maximize the probability that the trial would be successful" (Beutler 2004:119).[26] The maker must continually produce patient data to justify the drug's safety and efficacy profile, as well as to satisfy criteria for guaranteeing the drug's orphan status, which, in turn, leads to exemptions from normal price competition. From a company perspective, investigators worldwide play a critical role in affecting the "value of the clinical trial" (Finn 2006). Through the international Gaucher Patient Registry, the drug maker maintains control over knowledge of the disease, its natural history, and the evidence base related to treatment recommendations. "It cannot afford to permit the appearance of any doubt about its evidence base," I was told. "Doubt" of the sort introduced by Drs. Beutler and Zimran and the *Protocolos* team can sharply erode public confidence in the value of the drug.

From Dr. Picon's perspective, "translating evidence into practice without politics is impossible." The challenge now was to make practitioners in diverse worlds—medical, governmental, nongovernmental, and the courts— adopt the *Protocolos*, even in small parts. Members of the guidelines task force were hoping for a cascading effect—a new medical jurisprudence— that can serve as an antidote to medical overuse and, in some cases, harm. Resistance among Brazilian Gaucher doctors continued.[27] They argued that the guideline undermines best standards of care and that prescription at lower doses may cause patient harm. There is no consensus and the controversy continues.

The Clinical Research Unit

Every time I go to the hospital, I am struck by the multitudes of people waiting outside the facility. It is winter and generally cold there when I visit in July and August. The sick, old and young, are awaiting medical appointments or setting up future ones. They are joined by relatives and friends who usually sip *chimarrão* (a traditional strong tea) or chain-smoke—some are wrapped up in worn-out coats and brown and gray blankets. The scene conveys a sense of patience, neighborliness, and anticipation for the best treatment possible in the region. Many patients arrive from the interior in vans operated by municipal health secretariats. Because of the lack of specialized care in the interior, these "ambulance therapies," as they are called, transport the sick to the capital's overcrowded centers of medical excellence. They speak to the fragility and limits of the country's universal health-care system.

The Clinical Research Unit is located on the third floor of the east wing of the hospital. I first heard about Dr. Picon's enterprise from a medical geneticist working in a nearby medical genetics service, who had collaborated with my husband, João Biehl, on a study of gene-environment interactions in patients afflicted by Machado-Joseph's disease. The well-regarded service was participating in genetic treatment trials, particularly on expanding indications and uses of enzyme replacement therapies. Researchers were excited about the possibilities of finally offering patients something more than just an accurate diagnosis of their genetic ailments and immediate symptom relief. But they were also cautious about hyped claims of efficacy and about the high cost of lifelong treatments. And that is when Dr. Picon's name entered the conversation.

The Clinical Research Unit opened in 2003. It is strictly outpatient and semiotically transparent in its research-oriented purpose—the white monitoring rooms are spacious and comfortable, and there are provisions for intravenous infusions and laboratory exams. A proud Dr. Picon (who directed it until 2006) gave me a tour of the unit. "Here are the beds and equipment, the air conditioners, the TVs, computers, monitoring rooms, and telephones. It is all paid for by ANVISA [the Brazilian National Health Surveillance Agency]." He explained that the unit's origins are linked to the government's attempt to foster the production of generic drugs to deal with growing treatment costs. Since 1999, the Health Ministry had funded units for bioequivalence testing in several major universities. In other words, ANVISA wanted the unit "to test generic drugs and to demonstrate the efficacy and toxicity of older drugs. We are designing those trials for drug registration purposes."

The unit was also meant to attract industry-sponsored trials. Brazil's business-friendly environment, well-trained medical workforce, and pharmaceutical market growth made the country an attractive clinical trials destination. Trials were migrating to Brazil from places like Argentina, for example, after its 2001 economic collapse (though Argentina rebounded shortly thereafter). Indara Saccilotto, the unit's financial manager, told me that the federal government has been curtailing investments in research and medical infrastructure, and that university hospitals were struggling to find alternative sources of funding. The bioequivalence centers were a rare and much-welcomed instance of governmental support as academic research was increasingly industry-sponsored, which, though also welcomed, raised questions about local research autonomy as well as medical and financial conflicts of interest. I was told that 14 percent of the 550 protocols sent to the institutional review board (IRB) of the hospital in 2002 were sponsored by pharmaceutical multinationals. By July 2003, industry-sponsored research constituted 25 percent of the research carried out in the hospital.

Dr. Picon had established a partnership with the Pharmacy School of the Federal University for generic drug testing: "We do the clinical testing here and they do the laboratory work there. We are improving the university's technological infrastructure and ways of monitoring the quality of clinical trials." The challenge, he told me, was to reverse two trends: companies were testing generic versus standard drugs inside their own companies, and the majority of clinical studies were still taking place in outpatient clinics. Public accountability was at stake: "Investigational environments should be free of conflicts of interest. As much as possible, we want to create and interpret evidence free of such conflicts."

For now, the well-equipped and professionally run unit was underutilized and eerily empty. Few patients were scheduled, and few trials were actually under way—a medicine to treat rheumatoid arthritis, an insulin inhaler, a locally produced cough suppressant syrup, for example. It was not that the unit had difficulties in recruiting patients. "We post advertisements for trials inside the hospital, announce them on television, radio, and in newspapers, and we have a good doctor referral network in place," the administrator told me. The unit's high standards had raised costs, and it was not financially attractive to national generic firms eager for a quick monetary return in a high-risk business. "In other regions, companies take advantage of the public health infrastructure and of academic hospitals that do not have the strict clinical oversight offered here. In our unit firms have to pay for everything, including overhead costs. We keep tight financial control, but they get high quality in return."

A pragmatist, Dr. Picon was also using the unit as a platform for reordering research arrangements inside the hospital. He was working closely with the general administration to harmonize research practices and to develop a consistent framework of negotiation with trial sponsors. The industry tends to focus on individual physician-researchers for its recruitment, and "it limits the hospital's role to a functional IRB," Dr. Picon said. "It usually pays physicians directly, and I'd like this to change." The hospital wanted to use the new research facility to generate income to finance other research and infrastructure. In Dr. Picon's words, "We want to show there is a different way of negotiating with the industry, where the hospital can state its priorities and better regulate the terms of the contract." According to the unit's manager, "We are pioneers in setting up this kind of system, hoping it might be good for Brazil."

As we sat in one patient monitoring room, Dr. Picon recollected the recent history he was trying to reconfigure. He spoke about the "surge of trials coming from the North" in the wake of Brazil's 1997 compliance with the International Conference on Harmonisation and Good Clinical Practice standards. The ICH-GCP, as we have seen, is an international set of standards for testing experimental compounds and investigator conduct, and it includes guidelines for institutional review boards. As a transparent and investor-friendly mechanism, it makes data from new research sites transferable to regulatory bodies such as the U.S. Food and Drug Administration. At that time, Brazil established the National Committee on Research Ethics (Comissão Nacional de Ética em Pesquisa, or CONEP), to implement the guidelines for human subjects research in the country. CONEP is an advisory and educational body; it works in tandem with local ethical review boards, which maintain primary oversight responsibility. The hospital already had a fully functional review board, but many more were needed around the country. When the "surge" hit, these committees and procedures were not uniformly in place. For several years, I was told, such boards had a symbolic function, with very few resources and little power to issue independent judgments.

While the implementation of oversight mechanisms appeared to lag, companies were actively recruiting physicians into clinical research. The doctors I spoke with decried the seamlessness with which private-sector research began to merge with academic medicine and private practice. Dr. Picon referred to this time as a physician "buy-in" period. "You just have to follow the protocol and send off the data. It will be analyzed by people hired by the sponsor company, and you will be well paid for that job. And if you are a medical authority, an opinion leader in a valuable therapeutic area like cardiology or neurology, you are by extension influencing several hundred doctors at the same time."

Several doctors I interviewed agreed that independent medical judgment is seriously compromised. An internal medicine specialist periodically involved in industry-sponsored research, for example, referred to study protocols as "ethically ready. We are just supposed to follow the rules." He also questioned how drug efficacy was being measured and how biologically significant responses are actually defined. "Am I measuring something that is really important? Or is it just an epiphenomenon that is of interest to the trial sponsor?"

Another researcher pointed out that one of the most important services a doctor can provide to patients is the record of their clinical and treatment history. But trial contract provisions usually restrict investigators' access to data and a clinical trials database (Steinbrook 2005). The impact of data withholding is significant, this doctor argued, and can compromise basic principles of long-term medical care. "At the end of the trial," he said, "you will have tons of data on a patient. But the trial data from electroencephalograms, for example, are simply sent to the trial sponsors, and no primary or secondary data can be stored here. The information is proprietary, so we can't use it to track the patient's condition after the trial." If physicians could access these data, he reasoned, "We would have a better chance of knowing whether symptoms are a disease-related or a clinical trial–related adverse event. We would also be able to track the uses and abuses of our data."

I brought up these issues over data with the unit's financial manager. She stressed that more equitable contracts are needed to ensure scientific integrity and patient protection after the trial, "but this goal is not easily reached. There is a surplus of highly skilled professionals who will accept the given terms of the research contract, and it is a daunting task to reach consensus among investigators and sponsors over what is best from a clinical standpoint in the long run."

When a Country Is a Pharmacy

In the early twentieth century, a first generation of Brazilian public health activists described the country as a vast hospital. A century later, according to Dr. Picon and his collaborators, the country has become "a big pharmacy, with public health authorities at federal, state, and municipal levels spending more and more of their budgets on drug treatments for a progressively smaller number of people." Their work is a specific response to global pharmaceutical trends, and they engage in health politics at various institutional levels.

In her book *Territory, Authority, Rights,* Saskia Sassen writes of the erosion of collective structures that can hinder market logic. She argues that while the state helps to enable the expansion of the global economy, it does so in a context "increasingly dominated by deregulation, privatization, and the growing authority of nonstate actors, some of which assume new normative rules" (2006:269). The globalized research enterprise that I have been charting follows this trend. Old and new business actors outsource services, secure infrastructures, and make sure that legislative environments are in place and kept hospitable. Sassen sharply notes that the globalized state creates mechanisms of its own acquiescence in such commercial windows of opportunity: "This signals a necessary participation by the state, including in the regulation of its own withdrawal" (ibid.).

This regulated withdrawal, which also makes experimentality possible, favors economic interests over well-defined systems of protection. Sassen describes the withdrawal process as "extremely partial rather than universal, but strategic in that it has undue influence over wider areas of the broader institutional world and the world of lived experience, yet is not fully accountable to formal democratic political systems" (ibid.:270). In all, we see that the normative power of international law is being compromised, and sustained public debates, the hallmark of liberal democracies, are being severely compromised. If the country is a "big pharmacy," criteria for public investments in high technology and modes of risk assessment remain underarticulated.

In Dr. Picon's at times lonely campaign to implement national treatment guidelines, we can appreciate some of the politics of pharmaceutical globalization at both national and local levels, and how new forms of research and state authority under present conditions might be enacted. He and his colleagues are carving out a dynamic and contentious medical field aimed at reining in commercial interests and making academic medicine politically consequential. Through a number of activities at the Health Ministry, at the state health secretariat, and at the university, the group is attempting to contain the twin phenomena of pharmaceuticalization and judicialization of health and to work upon them.[28] These doctors are spearheading a statewide system of reference centers (*centros de referencia*), where the guidelines could be implemented for specific diseases and where drug value can be assessed on the basis of clinical outcomes.[29] Combining observational and epidemiological approaches, these centers are envisioned as extensions of Brazil's earlier infectious disease surveillance and control programs, which relied on a system of government-funded reference institutions (for tuberculosis, for example), that were designed for the monitoring and treatment of patients and assessment of optimal interventions. Accumulated evidence, in turn, informs national treatment guidelines and health policy.

In the *centros*, doctors chart what happens to real-life patients who are often much sicker than the highly screened ("biologically edited") subjects of clinical trials. Individual patients are carefully examined and their treatment habits scrutinized. Dosages are personalized, sometimes treatments are scaled back, and environmental and lifestyle factors are considered. A new patient database is in the making.

As I will show later in the chapter, these reference centers mobilize multiple parties and interests—health professionals, patients, administrators—and the data yielded are used to inform alternative pharmaceutical policies. Through the centers, the Protocolos physicians establish a knowledge base that balances the one of pharmaceutical representatives, lobbyists, and medical opinion leaders. They believe that "if you wish to solve your expensive-drug-treatment-public-health-problem," as Dr. Picon put it, "you will have to employ some of the steps we have been working on."

Dr. Picon was taken aback when I asked him how his biography had shaped his present work. "Is that important?" he asked. But as I insisted, he began to speak about his humble origins and his trajectory from the interior to the state's centers of medical excellence. In his recollection, it became evident to me that his understanding of science as political was also characteristic of a whole generation of progressive health professionals, deeply connected to struggles for democracy and social justice.

Paulo Dornelles Picon grew up in a small city on the Brazil-Argentine border, one of eight children in a working-class family of French-Spanish descent. His father was an auto mechanic, and the young Picon "grew up fixing cars and bikes. I fixed bikes for all my friends so that during the weekend we could go out." He also recalls making kites. "I used to build many and give one to each of my friends. We held contests to see which one worked best." His two older brothers were the first in the family to pursue higher education at the Federal University, and they became respected doctors. "Pedro is a pneumologist specializing in tuberculosis, and José is an obstetrician-gynecologist." He followed in his brothers' footsteps. "They were my role models, and they always supported me. But I didn't want to be a burden to them, so I worked hard to get fellowships. I also worked part-time to pay my own expenses."

In 1978, as a third-year medical student, Picon worked as a teaching assistant in clinical pharmacology. This was a turning point for him. He worked closely with Professor Lenita Wannmacher (known for her work with essential medicines at the WHO and at the Pan American Health Organization) and Professor Flavio D. Fuchs (still working in cardiology). His mentors were the first to introduce clinical pharmacology in medical curricula in Brazil, said Picon. "For the first time pharmacology would not be taught just as a basic science. It was not enough to look at the chemical structure or clinical efficacy of drugs."

"Flavio was Lenita's best student. He did his doctoral studies on hypertension. At the time, there was a lot of doubt about which medicines to prescribe. They have always been skeptical about the claims of efficacy." As a student, Picon joined this local effort "to critically evaluate evidence and to integrate mathematics, statistics, and epidemiology in the assessment of drug effectiveness in different populations." That is what critical clinical pharmacology is—"Big changes were under way in medicine and I caught that essential critical bug." It took about ten years for clinical pharmacology to be really understood by the medical community and to become a regular part of the curriculum. Today, says Picon, "medical students rank it the best course in their education."

Picon was a medical student in the waning years of the country's military dictatorship. "My colleagues and I protested in the streets. Soldiers threw tear gas at us. I never ran so fast. In the end, I had this mixed feeling of exhaustion, humiliation, and, why not, a bit of victory." He had always been a progressive as far as politics was concerned. He participated in meetings that led to the formation of the local wing of the Workers' Party, a party he supported initially, but he never became affiliated with any political party.

The graduation of the 1980 class epitomized reigning government-academy tensions. "University officials were appointed, and the professors were on strike, protesting against dictatorship and for better salaries. They asked us not to hold a ceremony because that would legitimate the status quo." From 1968 until 1979, there had been no official graduation ceremonies. It was a way for "us to say that we didn't endorse the military." Half of the class, however, "wanted the ceremony for personal and family reasons." Picon was part of the other half, who thought "we should be introduced to reality instead."

The young Dr. Picon did residencies in internal medicine and in cardiology. In 1981, as the president of the Association of Medical Residents, he led a strike for better working conditions and salaries. "We then went to Brasilia for the first time to lobby. I had a sense of what was going on in this big country, but it was only piecemeal knowledge." Fascinated with academic medicine, he embarked on a master's degree in cardiology. By 1987, he had taken up multiple professional activities: a private practice in Porto Alegre and teaching positions in pharmacology at the Federal University and at the University of Passo Fundo.[30] He was by now married to Patricia (a psychiatrist), whom he had met in medical school. The couple would soon have a son, now in medical school, and later a daughter.

"Ethics, not politics," made Picon eschew the more high-status field of cardiology. "I was invited to work in the department of cardiology, which is the most prestigious when it comes to research and recognition. I wanted to develop a more rationalized pharmacology, and that would be best done in internal medicine. Even though I was in a low-status department, my interests were there." His workload was immense, but he felt the need to keep practicing clinical medicine in addition to pursuing research and teaching. "Till today I have kept my private cardiology practice open, at least one day a week. The practice helps me not to lose focus on what is truly important. How much can I intervene in this patient's disease? What will be the outcome of my intervention, and how does this care relate to public health?" Here the politics of science cannot be ignored.

Since the seventies, a myriad of observers have critiqued the political and economic interests driving the exportation of pharmaceuticals—either approved, unapproved, or withdrawn to low-income countries, as well as unethical marketing practices and lax regulations concerning the selling of tonics, breast-milk substitutes, costly vitamin preparations, and luxury drugs.[31] There is a long tradition of the "dumping" of items before they are proven to be safe or effective (the global thalidomide disaster being the most famous example) and of government agencies giving in to pressures to spend scarce resources on extraneous or dangerous items.

Over the years, Dr. Picon witnessed major changes in health-seeking behavior among his patients. Better-off patients were now moving from doctor to doctor, treatment to treatment. By the nineties, "the import of medicines into the Brazilian market increased, and the industry began to influence prescription patterns as never before, not to mention all kinds of perks for high-profile doctors." As elsewhere, there was no sustained public debate about these changes in medicine. "I started to criticize what was going on, but I was sort of alone. I felt alone. Nobody was saying anything except for Lenita Wannmacher, who has remained a great source of support. I know that she has no connections to the industry, and we share the same perspective."

Politics and medical ethics came together in a new pedagogy. "We always had very sharp students. They had to read the scientific articles on the efficacy of new treatments and discuss them in class and in small groups. The *New England of Journal of Medicine* was difficult to get, but we made it accessible. We encouraged close scrutiny of methods, analyses, and results. Students wanted to outdo each other, and this was a healthy competition.

We discussed conflicts of interest the authors might have. This is one of the worst things that can happen in science." Dr. Picon and his group started to disseminate their evaluations to other residents and doctors. They began to think about guidelines for best prescribing and drug dosaging practices. By 2000, these local scientific pursuits had caught the attention of the country's Health Ministry.

A Public Health Experiment

In our discussions in August 2005, Dr. Picon voiced his frustration at how resistance to the *Protocolos* had bogged down its implementation. It was an uphill battle. He was juggling his research, teaching, and clinical practice with frequent consultancy work. Under the aegis of ANVISA, he was training physicians and policy makers in health technology assessment. He was also working closely with Fundação Oswaldo Cruz (the country's most prestigious medical research institute) on a Brazil-Cuba biopharmaceutical project to manufacture two high-cost medicines (human recombinant interferon and erythropoietin), which would be distributed through the national health system. He also worked as an adviser to the Pan American Health Organization on the rational use of medicines. In all these roles, Dr. Picon was crusading to make the new treatment guidelines operational.

Meanwhile, the testing of generic drugs at the Clinical Research Unit never really took off. The eerie emptiness persisted in the unit where we usually met. "We're saving a few local products here," Dr. Picon told me. He mentioned an athlete's foot treatment and used it as an example of the array of alternative medicines that are also part of the local pharmacopeia. "If this product goes off the market, the firm will go bankrupt." In the end, the efficacy study was negative, but the treatment decreased pain and itchiness, which meant that it could stay on the market for a few more years. To make things worse, foreign companies had been quick to step in to the generics market and were dominating it. "They have their own laboratories and testing sites," the unit's manager said.

Yet by no means was the Clinical Research Unit a failure. It kept playing an important role in the hospital administration's attempt to revamp its clinical research strategies. It had also become central to Dr. Picon's efforts to implement the *Protocolos*. He was now creating a network of disease-based *centros de referencia* inside and outside the hospital. These reference centers would gather patient data on the efficacy and safety of some of the guidelines, and the unit would be an operational base for their planning. Ideally, other states would replicate this pilot public health experiment (and some eventually did). A new patient database would be established (reports on diagnosis, treatment plan and response, laboratory follow-up, adherence, adverse effects, and dose optimization)—an active form of postmarketing surveillance in which data would be gathered on a drug's risks, benefits, and recommended use for a Brazilian population. These data would feed into a national database, critical for influencing pharmaceutical assistance programs. Physicians and patients were reenvisioned as critical partners in treatment. In the process, Dr. Picon and his team would endow their evidence-making enterprise with legitimacy and value for both patients and the public health system.

The first reference center would be focused on Gaucher disease. Dr. Picon thought that the Gaucher center was bound to be a success story. There was considerable international agreement over the efficacy of lower-dose treatments, and patients were eager to have drug access and quality care routinized now that imiglucerase was being purchased by the federal government. A success here could be used to galvanize local and regional support for creating other reference centers. Dr. Picon told me that it would be much more difficult to control widely prescribed and overused treatments, such as statins, but they were also on his agenda.[32] "If it is hard to obtain evidence and formulate best practices for a drug treating just a few hundred people, can you imagine what is going on with other drugs affecting millions of people? Where one single drug can be used for multiple conditions and at different dosages, or at different prices because there are two or three or ten companies competing for the same market share?"

About 5,000 patients are taking imiglucerase (marketed as Cerezyme) worldwide, including some 500 Brazilians whose treatment is paid for by the government. As mentioned earlier, treatment can cost more than $200,000 annually per patient, and the price has not decreased over the years. In 2007, sales totaled $1.1 billion, making imiglucerase a blockbuster drug (Pollack 2008:A1, A24). Dr. Picon and his colleagues first needed to gain control over the prescription and distribution of imiglucerase for the twenty-three Gaucher patients in the state of Rio Grande do Sul. The state's health secretary, Dr. Osmar Gasparini Terra, and other key officials supported these efforts. An outspoken public health physician and former state representative, Dr. Terra was ready to find ways to regulate the provision of high-cost medicines and to better administer public monies. And Dr. Picon was placed in the position of reviewing all treatment requests in the state. The next step was to ensure that medical genetics authorities would support the idea of a Gaucher unit applying the new protocol—experimental on its own (public health) terms. Doctors who had worked closely with Gaucher patients who were already coming to the hospital for their infusions were enlisted.

According to Dr. Picon, medical competence and the trust of patients were critical assets in making the Gaucher unit work. One of the clinicians, Dr. Melo, described himself as a lover of genetics. "I always wanted to study genetics. I like this combination of clinical work and research. The cases are rare, they are hard to understand, and you meet people from all kinds of backgrounds. It's not just the same pattern of disease expression. You have to study each case." Key here is the question of how to deal with particulars and differences: "to accept them and to tolerate them is very challenging." Just a few years ago, when this clinician studied genetics, treatment was a nonoption. "I studied more biochemistry than pharmacology." But with the advent of orphan drugs and their marketing, geneticists at the hospital as elsewhere began to engage trials and therapeutics. Always having a clear position helps this committed scientist to navigate the conundrums of being both a researcher and a clinician, and being part of an alternative medical collective helps him to keep nonmedical interests at bay. "In this world, one needs to make one's position very clear. If I say something, this is what I mean. I don't stay in the middle. What we do here requires teamwork."

With the infrastructure and personnel in place, the twenty-three Gaucher patients whose therapies were channeled via the state's health secretariat underwent a new medical review. They were "unplugged," so to speak, from the previous prescribing and data-collecting regime. Dr. Melo told me that "the manufacturer recommends beginning with the highest dose, and that was the norm until this new protocol came along. When we began the Gaucher center, we carefully evaluated all patients and readjusted their prescribed dosages accordingly. When necessary, we increased the dosages."

After six months of operation, the hospital's order for the number of vials of imiglucerase for the Gaucher patients began to drop—from approximately 400 to 250 vials per month. In 2005, the unit saved $1.2 million and started to collaborate with Gaucher centers in other states. As health secretary Osmar Terra put it, "We want to guarantee medicines for the population, but with the right dosages and proven efficacy."[33]

What Happens When Clinical Trials End

Brazil is an important site in the global cartography of genetic therapy testing. In the words of a senior geneticist whom I shall call Dr. Antonio and who works in a private hospital in the region, "We have centers of professional competence in this area, but that's not all. It is also a strategy of the industry because of Brazil's universal health-care system. The trial is a way of generating public demand for expensive treatments. There are good professionals in Argentina and Chile too, but the industry isn't going there as aggressively as it is here." Trials also engender medical migration: "Patients and families come from all over the country to participate in trials we run here. We even have people from neighboring countries where treatment access is not available and the legal climate is not as conducive as it is here."

The Gaucher treatment's global commercial success bolstered research into treatments for other related inherited disorders. There is no mystery as to why doctors and patients get involved here: "These trials deal with diseases that have been untreatable until now," Dr. Antonio stated. "We also know from previous studies that, in general, enzyme replacement therapies work, and this is encouraging. All patients will get treatment, even if at first they are on a placebo arm of the study." In order to carry out placebo trials, the company commits itself to providing the drug for all patients for two more years, Dr. Antonio explained. "The problem is when those two years are over, what happens afterwards? The doctor in fact has a great responsibility here. What I think is wrong is that the patient files a lawsuit against the state and the drug maker is off the hook."

Dr. Antonio and other researchers I spoke to were well aware of the important role that they and their patients played in these new experimental regimes. They gathered precious data and in the process facilitated a small but lucrative global market in orphan treatments. These physicians were open about the conundrums they faced as they entered this new experimental and therapeutic field. Neither industry pawns nor hero doctors, they said that some of the companies for which they did trials operated in highly ethical terms, while others, in the end, disappointed them. How could they best engage the possibilities opened by global clinical trials and use the new technologies (such as gene silencing and chemical chaperoning) to create relevant lines of inquiry and to provide the best possible care?

Dr. Antonio is involved in several industry-sponsored trials of biopharmaceuticals, and he detailed the problematic area of the clinical trials aftermath. "We have to deal with the problems that begin when the study ends, particularly the continuity of treatment and quality of care as patients return to their hometowns. Many patients return home where no health infrastructure is in place and no one is responsible for setting this up. Some struggle for continued treatment, others give up. These are practical and ethical problems and they are very difficult to solve."

Biotechnology companies are entering the field of orphan disease treatments, breaking new ground beyond the blockbuster model of drug development. For example, mucopolysaccharidosis (MPS) is a group of lysosomal storage disorders characterized by growth stunting, skeletal change, breathing difficulty, liver enlargement, and cardiovascular problems. The disease is not curable, but enzyme replacement therapy (ERT) used for Gaucher disease has proven useful in reducing nonneurological symptoms and pain. There are several types of MPS, and several Brazilian investigative sites are running trials (mostly Phase 2 and 3, as well as for drug dosaging) for companies that are competing for a share of this limited but promising market. Dr. Antonio was himself involved in one MPS study. The FDA had recently audited the site. "They looked at all of our documents, the consent forms, the ethical part, and the ways we carried out the trial, to make sure we didn't make up data. If we had bad results, it would have been the end for us." The unit was praised for its ethical compliance and the scientific integrity of its data-gathering practices.

Researchers I spoke to were exhilarated to be part of this new era of testing genetic therapies, but they also had reservations about their monopoly aspects. At industry conferences, I was told, speakers tended to present data in support of the "highest dose" paradigm, and there was little room for dissent—or doubt. One doctor told me that at a recent conference, a speaker presenting the case of a young girl insisted she needed enzyme replacement therapy for her condition. The therapy had recently been approved for marketing in Brazil, but there were no treatment guidelines in the public healthcare system yet. "What a coincidence. I had seen this girl in my office before. The family lives in another state, and their doctor said that she needed the treatment. The girl had a mild form of the genetic disease but was developing normally. The parents went for a second opinion and were told that she didn't need it. The family was at a loss over what to do and then came to me."

This doctor's clinical exam showed that "everything was okay" with the girl. He based his medical assessment on the available literature. "I told the patient and the family that at that moment there was no indication for treatment, but that we needed to carefully monitor her." Studies corroborated this assessment: ERT has proven effective only in patients with an intermediary form of the disease in question, and not a mild one like this girl's case. "If I am supposed to base my care on evidence, she should not be on ERTs now." The parents weighed how early treatment would impact their daughter's lifestyle and decided to forgo it because in spite of the girl's physical appearance, this doctor said, "she had a normal life now."

Yet for the speaker who advocated the manufacturer's position, the question of whether to treat was moot. He argued to skeptical audience members that there was no way of doing Phase 3 studies in all patients because of the rarity of the disease in question. He claimed that the treatment "had a preventive value even in the absence of trial data." He couched his argument in terms of the treatment's ability to "maintain the patient's normal appearance" rather than improve symptoms. This physician is concerned with how the effectiveness of new therapies is being "spun" for desperate patients and families and how this spinning "gets to the patient's ears." As he put it, "The companies say that all patients should be on treatment, but I don't think so. If you take five patients out of this pool, that's one million dollars."

Continuity of treatment weighs heavily on doctors who place their patients in trials for new genetic therapies. Several of the doctors I interviewed mentioned that when studies end, companies generally keep providing the experimental drug for some time, as part of either an extended-access or a compassionate-use program. "But all this is at the company's discretion," I was told. I also heard of how, in the posttrial period, some company representatives advise patients to file legal suits to access the new drugs that were tested on them. One doctor described the stress that some posttrial subjects face: "They are confused and scared for their lives. Many realize only in retrospect that the consent form they signed left them vulnerable. They feel betrayed by their doctors. And legal suits consume their time." There is a whole order of mobility and value making in global research that is demonstrably legal (guaranteed by regulatory and ethical norms and contracts). This order yields investigational environments that are highly productive for the industry for some time. Yet they also appear to effect potential harms for which there is no clear institutional accountability.

One could argue that the *centros de referencia* coordinated by Dr. Picon are trying to break the political-economic enrollment of patients and doctors in the drug's dominant value-making cycle. This southern reality both reflects and complicates Kaushik Sunder Rajan's analysis of the civics of global life science projects, specifically genomics and personalized medicine (therapy tailored to individual genetic profiles). Sunder Rajan argues that new diagnostic tests turn the healthy and insured American into a potential patient-consumer. "The potential market for a drug is enlarged from diseased people to everyone with purchasing power" (2005:24). This population of consumers-in-waiting is "indicative of future markets for potential therapies that the companies might develop and thereby consolidate value for these companies in a speculative marketplace." In contrast to this American scene, there are the experimental subjects of pharmacogenomic clinical trials in India who are not sovereign consumers as yet: "The worker's body becomes available to systems of capital—as well as to systems of science—as a source of value generation and as a source of knowledge production" (ibid.:27).

Such a binary scheme does not necessarily hold true in Brazil, where experimentation encroaches and thrives on a universal health-care system. Dr. Picon and others are dealing not necessarily with future but with present markets. And the poor are not only experimental subjects generating value via knowledge production, but they are also voracious consumers of treatments via the state. As clinical trials end (and companies no longer have the contractual obligation to provide treatment), the "trial" migrates into the public health sphere, so to speak. A perilous public health trial begins.[34]

"It is very difficult to put a continued treatment clause in the clinical trials agreement," one doctor told me. "Neither patients nor doctors are fully aware of this posttrial circumstance, and they are not prepared to deal with it." It is true that "companies often provide drugs for some time after the trial, but nothing obliges them to act consistently, and it all depends on whether the government will purchase them." And even when the government provides the treatment, the industry goes all out to monopolize prescription patterns and valuable patient data, I was told. Experimental subjects are caught in a crossfire between the hospital, the industry, and the state—all agencies that got them enrolled in the first place and, at this stage, dispute responsibility over long-term care. In some cases, out of necessity, trial cohorts become patient activist groups. As I learned from discussions, researchers and caregivers are left to devise tools (clinical, legal, and regulatory) to remediate the new medical realities and human rights challenges that arise when experiments enter into a posttrial phase. All parties know that patient value and therapeutic chances take shape within this microcosmic medical-political economy.

How can seriously ill patients be protected beyond the experiment?

The solution is political, several of the doctors I spoke to suggested. They said that Brazil needed a national policy that would codify stricter rules of protection in legislation. "I am firm on this point," a clinician told me. "If very sick people participate in a trial and a drug's benefit has already been established, then they should receive the treatment for as long as they need it, for life." Another researcher told me of an incident reported in a Brazilian newspaper involving an AIDS drug under study. The Health Ministry cited a company that had stopped supplying drugs four months after the trial in question had ended. In response, the company stated that CONEP, the National Committee on Research Ethics, had agreed to those terms.[35] While this researcher did not know the specifics of the case, he used it to illustrate how national agencies do not work in tandem and operationalize different standards for research and care. "CONEP does not require more from the industry." This is was just one example, I was told, of how the national regulatory institutions that had evolved alongside state reform and new global trade rules were largely pro-business rather than pro-citizen in their decision making (or lack thereof).

In 2006, an egregious case of unethical research hit the news.[36] The case involved a malaria study that had been suspended by the National Health Council (Conselho Nacional de Saúde) in December 2005. Since June 2003, some forty men in the northern state of Amapá who had taken the preventive measures recommended by the Health Ministry were systematically exposed to malarial mosquitoes. They were trained to capture mosquitoes before they were bitten by them. Twice a year, the volunteers let one hundred mosquitoes blood feed on their arms or legs. They were paid about ten dollars per day for the activity. The mosquitoes were then taken by the researchers for analysis. Several volunteers happened to contract malaria in a community that had had no cases in the recent past.

According to Brazil's largest newspaper, *Folha de São Paulo*, the study was financed by the U.S. National Institutes of Health and was coordinated by an American university in partnership with Brazilian research institutes. All the organizations involved, including CONEP, approved the study. There is an ongoing debate over whether English-language protocols had been adequately translated and whether or not key procedural information had been withheld and by whom.[37] According to Senator Cristovam Buarque, who presides over the Senate's Human Rights Committee, "There is no specific statute in the Brazilian legislation to criminalize those responsible for the use of human guinea pigs."[38]

Some academic researchers I knew were critical of the ways national agencies acquiesced to the inadequate terms of foreign trials. A culture of complicity among various institutions, I was repeatedly told, makes patient-centered research contracts difficult to craft. They wondered why CONEP had not yet advocated for lifelong treatment for patients on trials for life-saving medicines and felt that the agency should set a precedent. But there seemed to be no sustained nationwide medical debate or mobilization to specify legislation that would make posttrial treatment a provision in the clinical trials agreement. Moreover, local researchers generally accept the sponsor's terms and boilerplate consent forms, a physician told me: "I don't know if it is naïveté, but there is a concern that if people don't accept the industry's terms, then the company will take their research elsewhere." The fact is companies can abandon sites and move investments elsewhere. They use this mobility to create competition between investigative sites and, if necessary, to isolate more demanding sites, while decreasing the cost of a trial.

Local researchers are cornered—most of the time, I was told, they either give in to the terms of commercial research or stop doing research altogether. "The industry creates and manipulates this field of internal competition among investigative sites. So people end up compromising. Centers compete with each other for trials. They are left to make their own decisions, often against their own best judgments. They relinquish their power over matters of long-term protection and fairness because they want to do research," in the words of one researcher. More and more, at the end of trials well-intentioned physician-investigators face the reality that their capacity to care is impaired as treatments are not necessarily available. They are left with the difficult task of making sense of having agreed to carry out a trial that now, in its public health stage, might harm.

The Values Patients Bring

The Gaucher and other reference centers hint at what is at stake in global orphan drug business models and how the risks of experimentality can potentially be moderated. In seeking to recruit patients into a state-funded experiment of sorts, Dr. Picon's *Protocolos* team takes patient data out of industrial formulas (or proprietary international patient registries, for that matter) and reorients their value toward public health goals. Reevaluating prescriptions and dosages and personalizing treatment, members work to maximize outcomes and continuity and make high-cost medicine feasible. Dr. Picon says to physicians, "Your patients will get the drugs. You and the patients do not have to go personally to the health secretary and demand them. The flow of medication will be easier. And since you get the drugs and they flow more easily to you, you will give the public health authorities the real-life patient data. Patients get continuous treatment and we get valuable patient data. It's a deal."

But how is this situation different from patients' having to enter a commercial trial to get access to treatment? Is Dr. Picon complicit in a problematic form of rationing? I put these questions to him. He replied, "What is the other option? To not treat at all? We looked at data from other ministries of health in South America. Many of them are not buying the Gaucher drug. I was talking to an administrator from a neighboring country and I asked her, 'How can you tell me there is no Gaucher in your country, and only in Brazil? So your patients are dying and you are not doing anything?'" Prospects for health are shaped by the pressures of corporate monopoly; new public health experiments are needed in an effort to mitigate those pressures. The *centros de referencias* gather patient data and transform "the technical and formal content of [medical] work" (Timmermans and Berg 2003: 85). With access to patient data, the *Protocolos* team hopes to bolster the success of their postmarketing/alternative dosaging experiment, making the case for its replicability in other Brazilian states.

I further prodded Dr. Picon that a skeptic might say, "Okay, you are doing some good, reeducating doctors, saving public money. But is the state reinvesting this money, let's say, in prevention? What's so significant about saving money for the state?" He was candid about the difficulty of influencing the allocation of public monies. "No, no," he replied. "This money is already being used to extinguish another fire. The public health budget is always about extinguishing fires. I haven't seen change at this level." Solutions lie in changes to national laws on drug importation and distribution and in giving reformers and the health technology assessment community greater voice. Beyond money saved, the centers were leading to change at other levels. Dr. Picon insisted that "the patients are satisfied. They have regularity of treatment. They are happy. We know this from personal encounters and patient surveys."

In his view, the ability to monitor a patient over time is a social good in itself. And this practice is pedagogical: "doctors are being reeducated." Moreover, at the judicial level, lawyers and judges have access to "medical expertise," a new scientific literacy for a notoriously troubled court system decried by many as blatantly unjust. "Judges can ideally now cross-check information they are getting from patients and lawyers demanding treatments." In the end, this is not just about "making capitalism ethical," he said. These efforts must be scaled up and "must go to the national level and address research policy and intellectual property rights. We must come to that level. Pharmaceutical costs are off the charts." A drug pricing policy must be developed to foster "price control before registration" and "partnerships in technological innovation."

As Dr. Picon articulated a moral middle ground of political and medical maneuvering that goes beyond triage, I noticed that he was now employing,

if somewhat unreflectively, a new idea of the patient. In our previous conversations, patients tended to be cast as agents of legalistic and antagonistic
patient collectives. There was distrust, and many times I wondered why
needy patients and families had to be portrayed as nemeses or pawns of
companies when, in fact, they could be allies in the centers' alternative treatment regime. That kind of portrayal, I thought, seemed to have helped the
team to insulate itself from volatile and disease-centered patient politics
and to focus instead on a new technical and political solution: the reference
center. Recaptured by the center, patients were now described in the language of consumption as "satisfied individuals." Any language adjustment,
however modest, suggests how untethered citizens have become from public health institutions when it comes to their own health care and, more
broadly, the difficulty public health specialists have in creating solidarity
with patient populations, increasingly recast as market segments in a neoliberal state.

But what about the patients? I wondered how they had accepted becoming part of the Gaucher center's lower-dose treatment regime. "In general,
they accepted it very well," a physician told me in 2006. "Each patient is different from the other. Of course, some patients were concerned about dose
lowering, and at first they did not like the idea. But we didn't have a big
problem. Over time, all of them were happy with the care provided."

Yet the Brazilian Association of Gaucher Patients has criticized the low
dosing as a mere technocratic project of cost reduction. In December 2003,
the *Jornal Gaucher* insisted that "dosages should be defined by specialists,
not by a Protocol" and that subdosing was like "throwing money away because a patient will still have complications." The newsletter reported on a
patient who was doing well and, after a dose reduction (from 60 units to 22
every fifteen days), "had to be in a wheelchair and on crutches." After having the dose reset to 42 units, the patient "stopped trembling," but he still
had problems. "I have not been working. I have lost a year of my life," this
patient was quoted as saying.[39] There is another story in the same issue. The
mother of a teenage boy who was initially diagnosed and treated overseas
with the highest dose said he was now at the hospital. "We began the reduction, and he is being monitored." She defended the excellent results that
come with high-dose treatment but conceded that "so far, he is responding
well to half the dose."

I was curious about the subjectivity of patients and families partaking in
this public health experiment. Which pathways brought them to the center?
What was their rationale? How did they coordinate their own needs and

treatment outcomes? On one brisk but sunny winter day, I met Pedro Souza, now eighteen, and his mother, Lucia, a health professional. Pedro receives bimonthly infusions of the Gaucher drug at the hospital. In conversations with doctors, patients had often been cast in the generic terms of data collected or money spent or saved. But Pedro was engaged in a lifesaving medical routine. In their personal and legal quests, the Souzas conveyed a different genealogy of treatment access in which individual and collective lay actions are foundational.

Pedro had finished high school and planned to study advertising. He wore a fashionable T-shirt and jeans and had a quiet voice. "When I was child, I didn't understand what was going on. I recall all of a sudden going to the hospital, and my mom running after something. I didn't know why all that was going on," Pedro recollected. "But as I began to come more often to the hospital for treatment, my mom explained the disease to me and why I had to do this. She told me that the treatment was good for me." His mother said that being a health professional had made things a bit easier for her. "I am always updating myself. I had easy access to the medical literature. My husband had a harder time understanding Gaucher, but I could clarify things for him. To understand the disease was simple. The emotional aspects were the most difficult to deal with."

Pedro continued in his nonchalant youthful way, "I got used to the infusions. Sometimes I even forget about them and schedule something else for this time, and then I have to cancel it, what a drag. I could be doing something else and I have to stay still here. But I am used to it now. For a long time my friends didn't even know that I had Gaucher." This had recently changed as he had agreed to be interviewed by a local newspaper. Lucia explained, "There has been a lot of polemic about high-cost medicines and legal injunctions, and the article wanted to showcase a different side of the story. We agreed." Pedro seemed not to mind the publicity. He calmed his friends down, telling them that the disease "made no difference" in his everyday life, aside from the fatigue he experiences right after the infusions. "He is a very normal young adult. He dates, studies, and parties. But he has to take it easy with sports," his mother added. "It is great when technology can bring life to a patient and allow him to experience aging."

This was indeed a hard-fought and hard-won normality. Lucia was very proud of their having been "one of the first Gaucher families to have won a legal court injunction in the state of Rio Grande do Sul" and of helping to create the national and regional Gaucher associations. "Treatment is difficult in Brazil. We know that it is even more difficult in other countries. But in a few rich countries it is easier. In Brazil you must go out and fight. No one will fight for you. If you don't fight, you will have to wait longer or wait endlessly for others to fight for you." This caring and outspoken mother is painfully aware of the inequalities that are embedded in the judicialization of health care. "This is a very difficult situation. It is very convenient for us to have such an expensive treatment for Pedro. I work in public health and I know that most children do not have basic care. So there is this selfishness. You have care for your child and family, and you know that others do not have it."

Yet a humanitarian abdication of treatment access would not get to the root corruption that sustains this inequality, she said. "It is Brazil, but not just Brazil, that experiences this very shameful political crisis, of money being used to fulfill the desires of politicians. So how could I take up a humanitarian attitude and choose to forgo treatment for my son and share the money saved with the poor? I know that the money will not go to the poor." Lucia insists that people have to learn to fight for their rights at the most basic levels of health care. The resolution of the country's health crisis involves a combination of "high technology, education, and good management of public monies." The litigational culture that surrounds health claims also shields corporate and state institutions from taking fuller responsibility.[40]

In the early stages of their treatment battle, the Souzas literally administered public money. Their doctor put the family in contact with a lawyer "who had already gone to court successfully for families dealing with other genetic disorders." At the time, imiglucerase was not yet on the country's list of exceptional medicines, and the family resorted to the judiciary to guarantee treatment access. Local communities had also taken up Pedro's cause, and fund-raising campaigns were launched. "I have kept the posters people made. We even got donations from Brazilians overseas."

When there is a rare disease in the family, "one wants someone else who also experiences it to embrace you," Lucia said. "And we were directed to an adult Gaucher patient who lived in the interior. His treatment was paid for by a Brazilian bank. He showed us the vials, and, for us, it was like seeing a diamond, an impossible-to-get jewel ." But the family struggled on all fronts to get that jewel—"now treatment is a routine. If needed, we would do it all over again."

An English teacher helped Lucia to get in touch with the drug's manufacturer even before she won the court injunction. "The company representative advised me to contact a Gaucher patient association in Washington, D.C." A family in Rio de Janeiro who paid for the treatment, and who spearheaded efforts for free access, succeeded in putting the Souzas in contact with the drug maker. This family's lifesaving actions were intimately entangled in emerging local, national, and transnational medical fields. "We started to make contact with families all over the country. We exchanged information and the patient association made our struggles visible." This new type of treatment mobilization involved sustained activism and court battles. "After we won in court, the state wired the money to our personal bank account. We bought the drug directly from the company in the United States. We sent the company the money, and it sent us the drug by airplane. I picked it up at the Salgado Filho airport."

Pharmaceutical markets were going global, and soon this family's right to health would constitute a new market segment with the state acting as drug purchaser and distributor. Of course, Lucia does not recollect things in such straightforward terms. For her, there was still "too much bureaucracy" involved and not enough formalized procedures to keep imiglucerase flowing for the small but growing number of patients who needed the drug. "Other cases of Gaucher emerged, and soon the health secretariat realized that by buying in bulk they could save some money. These are people from all social classes. Gaucher is neither a disease of the rich nor of the poor." Families contacted each other and got organized. "We already had the national association. But we needed to set up a local branch to make sure that treatment would be continuous." Lucia explained that the drug's availability at the local pharmacy was irregular, and this caused much distress. "Three months of a regular flow and then two or three months without medication. Sometimes I went there and picked up the dosage Pedro needed, but there were no vials left in storage for the next patient in line. The treatment ran out for someone. At other times, Pedro needed ten vials, but there were only seven left."

"And what did you do then?" I asked.

"Waited and struggled." Solidarity was crucial. The Gaucher association decided that once a month one of the members would retrieve all of the prescribed vials from the state pharmacy and put them in a refrigerator. "We divided the doses among ourselves." When there was a shortage, the families consulted doctors and "even hospital ethical committees" to redose to minimally acceptable levels, making sure everyone got some. "We counted all that was left of the imiglucerase, and we set a minimum dosage for everyone. This was a humanitarian measure. We did this so that one would not get full treatment and the other none."

Interestingly, in these rough times, the Souzas never used their court injunction to favor their son's case. "This would have weakened our collective cause." The association opted not to file a class action suit against the health secretariat either, Lucia stated. "Our association always kept talking with the secretariat. We had support from public prosecutors working in child and youth welfare programs. Our aim was to ensure the continuous flow of therapies." The fact is that the political mobilization of the association stabilized treatment access. For Lucia, this victory is class inflected: "Richer families run the national association. They know the politicians and are closer to Brasilia. Since Gaucher became a national program, medication was missing on only one occasion."

As I listened to Lucia's account, I understood the Gaucher "low-dose experiment" as continuous with family struggles for treatment access and the new therapeutic market that took form through these struggles. One could argue that the *centro de referencia* is an extension of what patients desired all along and had begun to forge on their own: sustained access and quality care. It was also a remediation of the effects of new medical markets in which the state acquiesced, and this remediation spoke volumes about the limits and possibilities of governing global pharmaceuticals. As far as the experimentality of low dosing is concerned, "In my view, patients don't think of themselves as guinea pigs," stated Lucia. The collective practices of the Gaucher families (and not a technocratic protocol) seemed to have "prepared" them for adherence to this public health experiment. "With the reference center, we got our lives back. It is the struggle for access that is sacrificial." Now that there is treatment "for a lifetime," families can finally reengage ordinary routines. "That is what we gained here at the center." But things do not always turn out this well.

Information Asymmetry and Agency

In 2005, a group of doctors active in industry-sponsored research, and working in a research unit of another hospital, told me of a problem they were facing. They were conducting a Phase 3 clinical trial of a multicentered study to test the efficacy and safety of a new therapy for another Gaucher-related genetic disorder. The study of a genetically engineered molecule was sponsored by a Northern company and involved a dozen patients. The therapy had proven to be somewhat successful in stopping the progression of renal failure (a symptom of advanced stages of the disease). To the doctors' and patients' dismay, the company stopped providing the study drug in the third year of the study.

Like Gaucher, the disease in question is a lysosomal storage disorder. According to U.S. figures, the disease's prevalence is 1 in 40,000, and its treatment falls under the U.S. Orphan Drug Act. A faulty gene causes a deficiency of an enzyme; this enzymatic deficiency prevents the body from breaking down certain lipids, which then accumulate in the blood vessels of major organs. Throughout their lives, "patients complain of extreme pain and numbness in hands and feet," a clinician-investigator whom I call Dr. Lima told me. "Yet often they are not diagnosed because the disease is unknown to many physicians. Many times, their complaint of pain is brushed off as psychosomatic. Patients usually survive into adulthood, but they are at an increased risk for strokes, heart attacks, and kidney failure." Symptoms are heterogenous and are not age dependent. "A twenty-five-year-old might suffer from end-stage renal failure; a forty-five-year-old may just be starting on hemodialysis."

Before the discovery of the genetic basis of the disease, treatment was limited to symptomatic relief or palliative care. "When enzyme replacement therapy worked for Gaucher, then everyone starting paying attention to other enzyme deficiency disorders." Yet treatment costs are prohibitively high. The researchers I spoke to stated that the evidence for treating the disease in question with ERT is not as well established as it is for Gaucher. As Dr. Lima explained, "Gaucher is a one-cell disorder. We can deliver the enzyme to a specific cell like a macrophage and it will work. We see dramatic improvements no matter where the enzyme ends up. The spleen will shrink, the liver will get normal, and anemia will improve in a few months. But at least four different cells are affected by this related disorder. And these different cells are acting in different organs in different ways. It is very difficult to target all of them."

"We know that the drug works," a colleague added. "The questions are: How much does it work? When should we begin treatment? Should it be used for prevention, in childhood? But it is very difficult to test children. Some authors say you must treat. Others say more evidence is needed." These clinician-investigators were cautious about the hype surrounding treatment, and they were concerned about expectations that trials create. As they grappled with the force of this "biotechnical embrace," they voiced medical doubt and questioned what constituted best treatment for their stricken patients.[41]

Advanced-stage patients who had never been treated previously for the disease in question were recruited according to the study's strict inclusion criteria. A middle-aged man from the interior whom I shall call Inacio Santos told me that he had had symptoms of the disease since adolescence. In the early eighties, after he migrated to the South and attended college, an endocrinologist in private practice took an interest in his case. "When I had the money, I paid, and when I didn't have it, he saw me anyway." Inacio found a steady job as a public servant, and from then on half of his medical expenses were paid. "The doctor taught me how to live with the disease."

But Inacio also began to be studied as his doctor conducted medical research at a local hospital. "I went religiously to his office twice a year. I had to do all kinds of exams and biopsies; sometimes I went three or four times a year there." He treated himself with painkillers and an elastic stocking to take care of the swelling in his legs, he said. Finally, one day in the late 1990s, "the doctor called me and declared, 'I discovered what you have. It is genetic. There is no treatment yet. But people are doing studies, and some people from the hospital will contact you.'"

"What is research? It is something that can turn out right or not. It is risk. All in life is risk. I understand that quite well. And I decided to enter the study. The die was cast." Inacio was in his forties and knew that he had already lived "beyond the average of people with the disease. Most people with the disease at my age were already dead or had killed themselves." I asked him whether the study drug had improved the quality of his life. His answer was, "I have survived. I made a choice to enter the study. I could have chosen not to do anything, and maybe I would not be talking to you today. But there is no way I can know the actual impact of the study."

Inacio's trial subject agency evolved within a complicated web of expectations, calculations, and abiding medical trust. "We do many things based on trust. We trust in the hospital and the staff, whom we know are upright people. The only document I remember signing said that I was not responsible for paying the bill for anything. Everything they gave us, we signed. Company representatives made copies of the documents and, after all this, nothing [no treatment]. In the beginning, when we started the research and for two years they even gave me a full tank of gas. They gave me around fifty liters of gas to come here for the research."

As far as Inacio recalled, if the treatment worked, "those patients who were willing to continue were going to have the therapy for the rest of their lives." Inacio and other patients, he said, couldn't understand how a company that had been allowed to begin a trial could now be exempted from the legal responsibility to provide the treatment. "We exposed ourselves to the drug without knowing if it was or was not going to work. Some benefits the company had. We didn't die."

Back to the specifics of the trial. Members of the research unit were eager to secure the contract. In fact, two companies were bidding for their services, and the research team chose company A over company B. The first proposed an open study; the second proposal involved a placebo-controlled study, "which we rejected," one researcher told me. Moreover, company A's drug had shorter infusion times, and this was more convenient for patients. During initial discussions, the researchers argued for a contractual provision stipulating lifelong treatment for the subjects recruited, but this was not followed through on. As Dr. Lima put it, "The process of the trial is so specialized. Everyone's responsibilities are stipulated. Someone is in charge of the budget and coordination. Some people oversee patients and infusions, others take care of the data and of scientific papers, and so on." Tasks are compartmentalized: "And when you do that, something is lost somewhere."

Only when the company suddenly withdrew the study drug did the researchers I spoke to learn that their department head had given in to the company's demand to reserve its right to withdraw the drug at any time. This had even been written in the consent forms that the patients had signed. The drug had slowed the progression of renal failure in several patients, and the company had informally agreed to provide medication to all in the trial for some time. "If you stop treatment," Dr. Lima told me, "the loss of renal function will restart."

The clinicians felt helpless. People aware of the withdrawal suspected that the company simply wanted reimbursement from the state for the cost of the study drug now understood as treatment. Trial subjects were actually instructed about the specifics of their rights to health and on the pathways of legal action for treatment. Patients tend to be loyal to companies or brand-loyal, I was told. "It is gratitude for having been rescued from a scenario of disease with no treatment to a scenario of possible treatment. There seems to be an internal process at work here, a promise of faithfulness in exchange for medication." Whatever had led to the withdrawal of the study drug, the clinicians involved had no institutional and legal recourse. Some of the patients migrated to research units in other states; some were filing legal suits against the state of Rio Grande do Sul; and a few "call weekly asking whether we have gotten the therapy," one of Dr. Lima's colleagues told me.

Inacio and others were struggling hard to make sense of the new medical and legal dilemma they had been thrown into: trial subjects without experimental therapies and now engaging the judiciary at the state and federal levels. Who was responsible for treatment access? Who would pay? To whom should they be loyal? How were they actually doing medically? Who would help them?

Throughout our conversation, I was struck with the knowledge asymmetries Inacio conveyed and his capacity to manage so many unknowns at once and not succumb to desperation. Inacio struggled for a medical measure that could help him make the best decisions as to how to continue living. The experimentality that he had been thrown into took him way beyond the disease he once knew how to cope with. He criticized the fact that he and his fellow trial subjects did not have objective measures of their improvement—before and after the trial. I didn't get a clear sense from him whether he understood what the therapy might actually do for his condition, or whether he and other patients were aware of the open questions surrounding its efficacy. "I know that when I began treatment, I only had the problem with swelling. But now I also have hypertension."

Inacio wanted more information about the efficacy of the treatment he had received before deciding whether to participate further—in either the clinical trial or the judicial trial process. He was trying his best not to be overcome by the drive of having the drug at all costs. "We are without medication and we cannot pay for it." But before resuming "the research," he continued, "I would like to have all exams done so that I have a measure. Did my condition worsen or improve? I don't know this today."

As Inacio described how he and other patients filed a legal suit against the state to force it to provide the experimental therapy, I noticed a certain hesitation and shame in his voice. "I didn't say anything to attack anyone at the hospital. I am not part of a corruption scheme." He was not proud of having gone the legal route, and he did not idealize the power of a patient activist collective. "There was talk that the trial sponsor was having problems. A lawyer from the Brazilian Bar Association contacted one of the patients and he initiated a legal action. We followed. This was the only alternative we had. We were without medication. And according to the hospital, this medication was helping us."

As I mentioned earlier, members of the *Protocolos* task force were bringing their health technology assessment initiative to the attention of public health administrators; they were now scientific advisers to the state health secretariat and prosecutors. In 2006, one member described the outcome of the legal action Inacio and fellow patients initiated. A local judge had initially ruled in their favor, issuing a court injunction to make approximately half a million dollars immediately available for the group's treatment (this amounted to only a three-month supply of the study drug). However, a higher state court overruled the decision. For this scientist, this was an example of how the state was beginning to counter legal claims to overwhelmingly expensive therapies, but at the expense of someone like Inacio. A state prosecutor who knew of the case told me that "the higher court judge weighed the fact that the study drug was not yet approved in Brazil, and that the evidence of efficacy was insufficient." He added that "prosecutors also argued in terms of equity, showing how this money for a dozen patients could treat thousands of other patients also in need of treatment." A state court is making moves to hold the manufacturer responsible for the well-being of the plaintiff-subjects.

This prosecutor told me that there were about eight hundred new legal claims for high-cost medicine every month in the state. "This is a huge problem and the state has to create new capacities just to deal with this." He saw himself as a detective of sorts, having to become scientifically literate to be able to comb through the claims and identify prescription patterns and legal strategies. "We also check whether legal suits are being waged concomitantly against the city and the state governments. But, honestly, we don't have a system in place to track all of this." Another prosecutor expressed uneasiness in having "to constantly set the limits of what is really possible to deliver as far as the right to health is concerned." According to these lawyers, the state was "stretched to its limit" as it tried to administer citizens' human right to health as high-cost therapeutic markets boomed. "We have to find intelligent and balanced ways to regulate the right to health at a national level."

"Sincerely," Inacio told me, "I think that the state is the scapegoat here."

"What do you mean?" I asked.

For him, the state was not ultimately responsible for this pharmaceutical impasse. "The number-one entity responsible is the drug company. But if the research was allowed to come to Brazil, it was because someone at the federal level allowed it to happen. And who allowed it is coresponsible. The child was born and now someone must cradle it." Inacio says he "trusts everyone in the hospital," the people who "took great care" of him. But he also speaks of the hospital as being caught up in "a game that the nation allowed."

Uncertainty permeates all levels of this case. The case also reveals profound institutional and informational asymmetries and the limited negotiating ability that is at the base of the global clinical trial. The various parties involved in the trial conceptualized the benefits of their participation independently of one another, but one variable was left out: the harm that could occur if the experimental treatment were withdrawn. No party was systematically helping trial subjects to formalize their concerns and interests before and during the trial. The investigators I spoke to maintained that the value patients bring to the trial and to the drug remained unconsidered. Debates over patient protection are too often framed in narrow dualisms—informed consent versus coercion, or autonomy versus undue inducement—

and tend to skip this crucial moral and economic issue. Uncertainties pervade the aftermath of clinical trials as doctors struggle to make best standards of care available, while patients are hurled into a medical-legal vortex. Now, in retrospect, the clinicians I spoke to say that explicit guarantees for continuous treatment should, in fact, go hand in hand with informed consent.

Patients had been without medication for eight months, and they were now taking their case to the country's Supreme Court. Hospital administrators were prodding the company to restart the flow of study drugs (which it eventually did), and researchers were contacting other companies testing similar therapies. In the meantime, one of the researchers wrote a letter to the hospital's institutional review board, detailing the team's medical dilemmas and asking the board to be more proactive in the future. But, as these concerned clinicians noted, such changes need to happen in tandem with the introduction of broader patient protection clauses in national research regulation.

The travails of Inacio and his cohort mark the place where politics has failed to acknowledge the scope of risks that accompany experimentality's global business model. Public institutions play a vital role in arbitrating market logic, resolving the "impossibilities" that patients and well-meaning investigators face, and guaranteeing citizens' access to new medicines. Research of all sorts, both private and public, troubles the line between the experimental and the therapeutic. As the range of types of experiments grows, the character of medical care in both rich and poor contexts is changing and new instruments for the right to health need to be devised. The life of the *Protocolos Clínicos* offers a crash course in the institutional resistances and human hopes surrounding new medical technologies. Their existence challenges public policy experts in other low-income countries to "deal" with the avalanche of high-cost medicines. Indeed, science cannot escape the reality of politics. But a different sort of scientific politics can optimize the uses of given medicines and engage the complexity of their outcomes, and provide tools for what comes next. In the conclusion, I consider recent efforts to bridge clinical research and the global right to health. How can commitments to distributive justice unsettle and animate ideas of innovation, both technological and social?

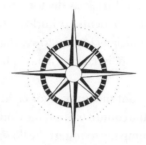

THE FUTURE OF
GLOBAL MEDICINE

Scientific Evidence and Value

Clinical research is essential to pharmaceutical globalization, but it also presents many challenges. In this book, I have explored the organizational cultures that make offshore clinical trials possible, the interests they serve, and the ethical and legal precepts that govern them. I have also probed, particularly in the pharmaceutical frontiers of Eastern Europe and Latin America, the context-specific calculations by which particular biological resources are sought and experimental groups configured. I charted the ways the private-sector research enterprise becomes a worldwide network, drawing from and thriving in public health institutions, and how governance and medical care occur in global but varied investigational contexts. In Poland and Brazil, I questioned the meaning and implications for subjects of the exponential growth in drug trials, and asked about how subjects are protected, how scientific integrity is ensured, and about the value patients bring to clinical trials and, ultimately, to the value of drugs.

Clinical trials account for the lion's share of research costs, but the public has known very little about the kinds of trials, the people involved as subjects, or the infrastructures, conditions, and risks characterizing the experimental context. While more detailed country- and region-specific assessments of globalized research are emerging, our understanding of its scope remains limited owing to the "incompleteness of records of some trials and its US-centric nature" (Thiers, Sinskey, and Berndt 2007:13). A largely uncharted field of global experimental activity has been taking form over the past decades—sometimes beyond what established regulations can control or even keep track of. Current institutional ideas about patient protection are narrowly construed, and the dominant research paradigm underhypothesizes drug safety. Biased protocol designs can "engineer up" the success of trials. And a procedural form of ethics that facilitates the portability of data can hide contextual uncertainties. Decentralized and diffused, this experimentality has thorny and sometimes contradictory value consequences. It may contribute to health benefits, but in leaving behind partial scientific evidence, unforeseen harms, and new medical and legal realities, it may also carry the seeds of its own failure.

In 2007, the inspector general of the U.S. Department of Health and Human Services published a report highlighting the Food and Drug Administration's failure to provide adequate oversight of clinical trials in the United States. The FDA, the report charges, grossly underinspects clinical trials sites and is "unable to identify all ongoing trials and their associated trial sites." Further, "uncertainty of timing and lack of coordination impede FDA's ability to conduct . . . inspections" (OIG 2007:ii). Moreover, the FDA's guidance and regulations "do not reflect current clinical trial practices" (ibid.). Writing in response to this scathing report, bioethicist Arthur Caplan asks, "How can it be that we know how many pigs, frogs, rats and monkeys are used in research and who uses them without knowing what is going on with respect to human beings?" (2007). The inspector general's report recommends improving information systems, creating a clinical trials database and an institutional review board registry, and establishing postauditing feedback mechanisms. Caplan agrees that such technical fixes are long overdue, but notes that without political will and adequate funding from Congress, the FDA will not be able to remediate its failings or close loopholes.

Clinical research is now a worldwide data-making enterprise, one that has arisen in tandem with new drug approval criteria and incentives, regulatory oversight, evolving trade rules, and related business opportunities. Contract research organizations implement globalized research on behalf of the pharmaceutical and medical device industries. CROs instantiate experimental environments in countries that make their diseased populations available for research, and that compete for a slice of the global clinical trials market. Of particular interest are countries with solid medical expertise, an efficiently working and pro-industry regulatory regime, and market viability. In the cutthroat world of clinical research, CROs claim to reinsert rigor, safety, and accountability into clinical research. Their niche is the very idea of a self-regulating market. Yet in practice they often also export problems, such as those noted in the Department of Health and Human Services report, that remain insufficiently addressed in this country.

In this book, I have considered the new geographies of pharmaceutical capital and power that facilitate experimentality—a convoluted reality whose quality is not solely dependent on standardized modes of compliance or procedure, but on how commercial, regulatory, and scientific priorities are set both here and abroad. In revealing the offshored dimensions and accelerated temporality of this phenomenon, I have raised questions about the adequacy of norms of protection that are in place in the United States *and* internationally, how they are modified, how they vary from place to place, and how data are strategically manufactured and, at times, strategically withheld. The benefits deriving from globalized research are arguably uncertain, and its risks are unevenly distributed and its costs, unjust. For the competitiveness around human subjects to flourish, patent-related agreements and harmonizing guidelines had to be in place to ensure the easy transferability of data. The same system that keeps investigators adhering to a preset form of ethics also works to define and protect patient data as intellectual property and to downplay research-related harms, such as those that take shape against a background of health crises, variable levels of state protection, medical conflicts of interest, and uneven bargaining powers.

The ability to proactively account for harm is becoming a unique selling point for an expanding trials industry that must deal with the risks the pharmaceutical industry defers. CRO scientists are specialists in this regard, but they are also generalists who toil in a reigning paradigm of expected failure. In the cartography of drug development, the world is becoming a network of interlocking research and data-producing fields, rescue countries, treatment-saturated and "naive" sites, and future markets. Informed public scrutiny and sustained political efforts at both national and international levels are required to ensure that the subjects of trials derive some benefit (in the form of posttrial treatment) for commodities that are slated for the well-off. We also need to ensure that consumers do not become unwitting experimental extensions of engineered trials that bring ineffective and unsafe drugs to the market.

Internationally, efforts to bring about the kind of research transparency and better information systems advocated by the inspector general of the Department of Health and Human Services are already under way. The World Health Organization's global clinical trials registry collects information about ongoing, completed, and published trials. Country- and region-specific registries are evolving and are feeding into a central registry. Yet, by themselves, they cannot capture how clinical research is organized as an economic activity nor how it becomes, if momentarily, a "normal" part of health delivery or a morally sanitized social good. Auditing and oversight must be coupled with innovative legal strategies that would make pharmaceutical companies responsible for trial and drug safety in a direct and timely manner. Such multifaceted strategies serve several public health objectives: disclosure of risks, deterrence of harmful practices, and adequate compensation for individuals and health institutions.[1]

As I documented in Poland and in Brazil, in ailing health-care systems, resources-strapped administrators and researchers find the possibility of introducing clinical trials attractive. So, too, do desperate patients who otherwise would go without treatment or better-quality follow-up care. The drug industry is quick to argue that in launching trials it is providing valuable treatments at its own expense to people who may otherwise never get them. This may be true, but in a limited and circumscribed way. How notions of well-being become increasingly tied to access to approved or experimental drugs is a complex process. In making doctors familiar with new medicines and fueling patient demand, clinical trials also become powerful marketing tools and can significantly alter local and public health care priorities. Neoliberal medical globalization transfers human rights and justice concerns away from traditional public domains to the privatized body of the atomized citizen.[2] Patient groups mobilize for treatment access from drug-purchasing states. Their lives are consumed by a market-mediated biological citizenship. Continuity of treatment and control of patient data by trial sponsors—points generally not anticipated in contracts and not articulated in informed consent forms—are pressing issues for regulators, researchers, and informed patients and their representatives to address. Likewise, new technology assessment programs that can independently assess the value and innovativeness of new medical technologies need to be strengthened so that financially strained public health institutions have a reasonable chance of promoting responsible and sustainable health-care delivery rather than succumbing to a pharmaceuticalized form of care.

In my efforts to chart the experiments, ethics, and aftermaths of industry-sponsored research, I encountered local scientists who were working to reverse some of the damaging side effects of an emerging global research and development footprint. I strove to make their concepts, pathways, and politics visible in this book. Scientists and physicians in southern Brazil, for example, are breaking the cycle by which trial participants, both patients and doctors, are enrolled as uncritical advocates and brand-loyal consumers of new high-cost drugs. They are redefining the dominant value regime of global pharmaceuticals and subjecting the new private/public processes that have strangled basic health care to an innovative evidence-enhanced clinical science. Moreover, they are, not without controversy, integrating their findings into regional and national health systems and influencing legal decisions.

How is the pharmaceutical industry dealing with greater scrutiny in the United States and internationally? What is its place in the global health mosaic? In the remainder of this conclusion I place the southern Brazilian initiative in dialogue with more visible international initiatives that are working to narrow the gap between clinical research and public health and to promote access to lifesaving medicines for the neediest. I also address the role academic medicine could and should play in the development of these international and domestic efforts.

Drugs as Public Goods

"Creating drug markets is getting so complicated," one professional whom I call Tom told me in 2006. The fifty-year-old economist with a medical degree works in the global pricing department of a pharmaceutical company on the West Coast. Pricing drugs is getting trickier, he says, as "almost every country in Western Europe has its own criteria for deciding whether a drug is valuable to them or not. It's crazy. When you deal with the regulators, they say they want to see, let's say, a 30 percent improvement for this cancer drug over the existing one, and if we can't meet their criteria, forget about market access there. They'll never approve it."

Tom works closely with research and marketing teams to place a value on each new drug his company produces. He assesses the specificities of pricing and funding in the country (referred to as a "market") in which the drug will be sold. He then proposes a global pricing and reimbursement plan and a country-by-country pricing strategy. Tom readily admits that the often exaggerated claims of marketers can undermine sound judgment on pricing and reimbursement. He also told me that the method of health technology assessment, with its emphasis on evidence-based decision making in health care, is gaining popularity in government settings and complicating pharmaceutical companies' global market access.

In an attempt to contain costs, national payers (as governments are called), particularly in Western Europe and Australia, are promoting generic drugs and becoming much more scrupulous in drug-effectiveness claims. They are demanding more data about a new drug's risks and benefits for their specific patient and consumer populations as a condition of market access. In the wake of regulatory scandals, including the FDA's delayed acknowledgment of the risks of several new drugs, government officials are more carefully scrutinizing the potential financial and medical hazards of new high-cost treatments. They are demanding more transparency and better financial arrangements that reflect this pharmaceutical unknown. With these new risk-sharing agreements, governments and insurers can effectively exact a refund from a drug maker on a drug that does not live up to expectations. From Tom's perspective, such "pay-for-performance" agreements are ambiguous, prone to fluctuation, and financially risky: "Five years down the line we may be dealing with new administrators who might have a totally different set of expectations or ways of measuring outcomes or value."

Value is the word of the day. A week after I spoke with Tom, I spoke briefly with his colleague Frank (a pseudonym). Having worked in Asia and Latin America before taking over as the director of worldwide pricing, Frank is a master of the art of drug pricing. In discussing its principles, he maintained that the benefits of pharmaceuticals are public, not private, in nature. "We don't produce profit, we produce *value*," he insisted. His notion of value was, of course, monetary, but the vague sense of the pharmaceutical as public good that permeated his understanding of value was also strategic. It allowed this pricing guru to mobilize more allies and resources in resolving the global market access problems that his company faced.

The value of a drug does not lie solely in the therapeutic functions of new molecules or of modified ones, nor does it depend on novel modes of delivery. Drug value is highly charged, economically and politically. It must be negotiated with multiple partners outside the pharmaceutical pricing complex. In affluent countries, governments and private insurers are "experimenting with new ways to create cost-justified payment systems for medical treatments" as a condition of market access (Pollack 2007a:C1). And the industry is refining its own value discourses in response to these political trends. The pricing experts I spoke to were fluent in a discourse of value, particularly around access and equity, and turned it into an "ethics-informed" market-making strategy. "*We* are making access possible," Frank contended. Treatment access becomes a value in its own right—even if the prioritization of a certain treatment is unclear or the means of access are not specified or are not applied invariably. This valuation can build political support and meet economic goals. Such value discourses do not, however, engage the failure of the market to advance a socially optimal level of drug research and development.

Vast inequities remain between affluent countries and those too poor to afford high-cost medicines. A growing number of activists and academic scientists are pushing for those inequalities to be considered and factored in to drug development and valuation.[3] Frank told me that the pharmaceutical industry was adapting to the human rights and social justice frameworks that had successfully politicized access to treatments and health care in the recent past. Referring, for example, to the ongoing struggle over continued access to state-of-the-art antiretroviral therapies in Brazil, he said rather bluntly that his company had co-opted the activist role: "You don't need the activists, just buy our drugs."

We live in a time in which the capitalization of markets and "markets in civic virtue" operate in parallel and frequently coalesce. As anthropologist Paul Rabinow notes, the challenge for social scientists is to identify instances of this conflation and "to investigate how 'capital' from one market is converted into 'capital' (or advantage) in another" (2003:26). Call it a new pharmaceutical modus operandi. As companies market the idea of the pharmaceutical as a public health good, they are indeed entering into new partnerships with development agencies, national health ministries, philanthropic institutions, multilateral agencies, and nongovernmental organizations to address the access gap. Which alternatives does this proliferation of partnerships and conversions of capital make feasible? What remains unaddressed?

Global Health Markets

Public-private partnerships come in various forms, have multiple interests, and create new norms for institutional action. They have stepped in to fill public health voids in places where national systems and markets have failed or have been absent altogether.

One of the earliest initiatives is Merck's partnership with the Task Force for Child Survival and Development, through which the company donated ivermectin (Mectizan) to fight onchocerciasis (river blindness).[4] Another example involves efforts by Pfizer in conjunction with the U.S. President's Emergency Plan for AIDS Relief (PEPFAR). Pfizer loans medical as well as financial and organizational management experts to help local NGOs and ministries of health support health systems and "deliver an uninterrupted supply of high-quality, low-cost products that will flow through a transparent, accountable system."[5]

These efforts have afforded unprecedented access to lifesaving drugs. Yet some critics have argued that the focus of many new large-scale treatment initiatives has been narrowly conceptualized and is overly technology and commodity centered; that is, it is missing an understanding of local cultures and health systems and does not sufficiently promote prevention and much-needed improvements in people's basic living conditions.[6] Some contend that corporate philanthropy is a good public relations move, offsetting public criticism of the depth of the pharmaceutical industry's political influence and the opaqueness of its drug-pricing practices. Moreover, partner companies can use these initiatives to gain a foothold in developing-country markets, to influence national drug policies, or to improve drug distribution networks. Others in the global health field argue that large-scale treatment initiatives have shifted attention and resources away from basic science—this is where issues of drug resistance and new therapies for neglected diseases can be targeted and where the quality of global health could be dramatically improved.

Whatever differences there are across corporate, activist, and public health agendas, the new rubric of "value" appears to reconcile these differences and folds them into a new ethos of collective responsibility.[7] Arguably, participants can become immune from critique as they point to dire global health statistics and their nonoptional duty to act (that is, to partner). So far, few, if any, institutions are in place to monitor and to promote accountability in this burgeoning and somewhat disordered "public goods" field.

Indeed, there is considerable confusion about how the new players and initiatives fit together in a "global health architecture" (Cohen 2006), and there is ongoing debate over whether such an architecture can actually be constructed and by whom. The interests and concerns of donors, not recipients, tend to predominate, and the operations of international organizations tend to reinforce existing and unequal power relations between countries. For instance, the long-term sustainability of some of these initiatives remains uncertain, and crucial questions linger: How do we politicize health-seeking among the poorest?[8] How do we integrate governments and national health systems as effective partners in global health?

Anthropologist and legal scholar Annelise Riles has argued that novel transnational formations (such as those she studied promoting women's rights) often operate beyond formal contracts and organizations (2000). Networks and partnerships deploy a universal lexicon and are diffused and sometimes chaotic in form. They are both fragile and powerful means to mobilize information, allies, and resources. In this mode of global "postpolitics," much is sidestepped. We need new analytic frameworks and institutional capacities that can address the fragmentation of efforts in global health, as well as broaden social impact and keep national governments and donors accountable in the long run. Moreover, new public-private initiatives should not divert the attention of activists and policy-makers away from the need for comprehensive reforms in drug pricing, patent law and intellectual property regimes, and health-care infrastructure.

For better or worse, pharmaceutical markets are increasingly conceived and operationalized as global health markets. This development dovetails with the phenomenon that I have been charting: with research offshoring, traditional modes of patient protection are being challenged, while experiments themselves are being touted as *global health goods.* As the rhetoric of value flourishes, the global experimentality this book explores continues to spread. Meanwhile, regulatory agencies could do better in detecting inadequate research practices and ensuring data integrity and drug safety beyond the trial period. When the focus of the experiment is on portability of data, the uncertainties of its context- and patient-related variables can be engineered out. And this in itself, as some of the CRO scientists I spoke to suggested, is a risk that may show up later as harm. The scientific integrity of this experimentality is *not* a given. It has to be periodically checked and optimized. This optimization is itself a commercial specialty for contract research organizations and their overseas associates. Industry and academic scientists testify to the pitfalls and question the public value and safety of the resulting medical commodities. Ultimately, this experimentality underwrites a research agenda that does not necessarily provide the most valid and relevant medical outcomes, and it introduces added risks. Whether they work for the clinical trials industry as scientists or as independent-minded academics, they reaffirm the critical need for a more socially responsible and scientifically rigorous approach that can value patients and make globalization "good for world health" (Pogge 2007).

Indeed, industry research priorities continue to sustain the so-called 90/10 research divide. That is, only 10 percent of drug research is committed to conditions that make up 90 percent of the global disease burden.[9] Anchored in a monopoly-patent regime and predicated on a blockbuster drug-development model, this arrangement is "morally deeply problematic," writes philosopher Thomas Pogge (ibid.:2). Pogge argues that huge industrial R&D investments in the commercialization of profitable but often non-essential medicines in the developed world might not be problematic on its own terms. But, he points out, juxtaposed with the global disease burden, these R&D priorities make evident the limits of innovation in private-sector research and expose the dire need to find new ways to develop and invest in science that has broader applications in public health.

Serious attempts to rethink drug development as a "public-good strategy" are under way. Pogge, for example, proposes a reform plan that would change "existing rules for incentivizing pharmaceutical research" and that would recruit scientists into a sweeping global health effort, providing them with stable and reliable financial incentives to address underresearched diseases affecting the poor (ibid.). Unlike the government-sponsored exclusive marketing incentives underwriting the development of new drugs, including high-cost orphan drugs (see chapter 4), this new family of incentives seeks to address what Pogge and others consider to be the real orphans: biomedical innovations that are not being developed because they are unprofitable.[10] More public and private funds are needed for health research into problems such as diarrhea, malaria, tuberculosis, and pneumonia, which, combined, account for 21 percent of the global disease burden (ibid.:7). Pogge calls for the establishment of a "suitable measure of the global disease burden" and methods of weighing the contributions that new treatments make to its reduction (8). Innovators in the field of essential medicines would be operating under a different drug-development patent regime and would be rewarded with market share.

Here, too, one could argue, market and activist values coalesce. What is being articulated is a market-based approach to achieving global health equity. Once taken as the nemesis, the pharmaceutical industry, with its enormous capacity, capital, and technology, has to be reckoned with as part of the means to bring about social progress. Pogge's model would not affect existing patent regimes covering nonessential drugs (for hair loss, acne, and impotence, for example), since affluent people, he argues, will most likely pay high prices for them regardless of whether the ailments they treat contribute to the global burden of disease. While this "public-good strategy" does not reckon with the pragmatics of the right to health in the field of high-cost medicines, it makes headway in retooling current international trade rules and in broadening the social mission of for-profit research.

Innovation

In diverse quarters, the search is on for making distributive justice central, not subsidiary, to new lines of innovation. Working in the field of genomics, Robert Cook-Deegan and colleagues are promoting the specific idea of a "science commons" that would make research findings available to public and private stakeholders at little or no cost and that could be used, managed, and owned. These academic scientists argue that many of the benefits of discoveries about health and disease "come not from drugs, vaccines, or medical services, but from individuals acting on information" to create social returns (Cook-Degan and Dedeurwaerdere 2006:303). Publicly available information, for example, allowed the scientific community to mobilize and to epidemiologically prove the harmful effects of smoking, which led to alternative control strategies and ultimately to disease reduction. In the case of penicillin, the government and the private sector worked jointly to create an affordable and accessible drug. These examples show that true biomedical innovations can transcend the value patents afford. Innovation should be broadly conceptualized in the life sciences and global health. "Continued institutional experimentation" is required. "Diffusion of knowledge and the exploration of new lines of innovation depend on creating institutions for collective action" (ibid.:313).

Consider the work of the Institute for OneWorld Health (iOWH). Founded in 2001 by Victoria Hale, a former FDA drug evaluator and Genentech pharmacologist, iOWH is the first nonprofit pharmaceutical research company.[11] Dr. Hale and colleagues are working to develop new drugs and to recycle old ones on the basis of global health needs rather than a financial calculus. Working with committed scientists in both industry and academia and with philanthropic investors, iOWH addresses the neglected infectious diseases affecting people who are too poor to make up a market attractive to private-sector R&D investment. The business model is as simple as it is pragmatic: identify undeveloped and unprofitable drug candidates, secure intellectual property rights, test them preclinically, and then run clinical trials with invested communities and seek regulatory approval for their licensing and distribution in countries that would benefit most.

In 2006, iOWH received approval for the use of paromomycin to cure visceral leishmaniasis, a deadly parasitic disease spread by the bite of infected sand flies. Annually, leishmaniasis contributes to the death of some 60,000 people living in tropical and subtropical countries. Paromomycin was an off-patent antibiotic. It was shelved, and trials were needed to show its antiparasitic activity. The Bill and Melinda Gates Foundation seeded iOWH's paromomycin project with a $10 million grant. In collaboration with the Special Programme for Research and Training in Tropical Diseases of the World Health Organization, OneWorld Health concluded a Phase 3 clinical trial of 667 patients from Bihar, India, in 2004. The Indian government approved injectable paromomycin, and the drug is being produced locally. This first success story legitimated iOWH and its concept of social entrepreneurship.

OneWorld Health's efforts resonate with the work of physician-anthropologist Paul Farmer and the organization he cofounded, Partners In Health. PIH champions access to health care as a human right, and it partners with poor communities to combat disease and poverty. Farmer and colleagues have been challenging "morally flabby" cost-effective models according to which the goods of modern medical science are impossible to deliver in resource-poor settings, and they have innovated treatment protocols with community-based support.[12] PIH's pilot projects in the slums of Lima, Peru, and squatter settlements in rural Haiti have debunked the conventional wisdom that multidrug-resistant tuberculosis and AIDS could not be treated in these settings. Both initiatives have been expanded and adapted in other affected countries.

For Farmer, as for Hale, standards of medical care and of research must be approached from a transnational perspective. Neglected people and their plights should inspire pathways of medical innovation, not drive them away. People-focused, Partners In Health and iOWH experiment institutionally with their commitments to distributive justice, and in their efforts they expand the realms of feasibility and shape new norms of intervention. Here medical change is not solely market determined, and the role of the public sector in health delivery is acknowledged and strengthened. These models of biosocial invention do not diminish the urgent need for a well-coordinated infusion of public and private investments in basic science that has global health relevance. For this to happen, we need alternative international frameworks for pricing and intellectual property, frameworks that address the needs of the developing world and thus provide a more cogent social imperative.[13]

This book has documented the existence and the effects of a troubling and proliferating trend: the use of vulnerable patients as experimental subjects. While goodwill and giving flourish via global health initiatives, ethical variability in clinical research continues unabated. Once at the periphery of global trade, local health systems have become cogs in the outsourced research enterprise. The clinical information obtained engenders profit for companies, but local returns are fragmented and short-term and social benefits are arguably minimal.

Private-sector research thrives on the public sector, and the public sector is altered in the process. The integration of clinical trials in local institutions is often accompanied by the conceptual reduction of health care to drug delivery at both national and international levels. Massive expenditures on prescription drugs overwhelm public health-care providers. Prevention and infrastructural reforms become ever-lower priorities. At the nexus of market-driven medicine, neoliberal state reforms, and human rights discourses, citizens are reduced to their own private hyperindividualized skirmishes for treatment access. As is evident in Brazil, there is no end to the number of patients going to court, staking their claims for access to new and high-cost medicines that are not yet included in pharmaceutical programs. In the southern state of Rio Grande do Sul, for example, new judicial claims have soared, raising questions over how states determine and guarantee the availability of new medicines and the human right to health. As demands for pharmaceutical access overwhelm prevention programs, "understanding what is happening in Brazil right now is of great value for countries that will soon face this avalanche."[14]

The prospect of a worldwide "avalanche" of such skirmishes over high-cost drugs raises vital questions about standards of care and public health priorities and equity, and these unsettling realities of pharmaceutical globalization unfold in tandem with the more visible and exciting new worlds of global public-private health. Scrutinizing and enhancing the evidence base of new high-cost medicines, creating alternative treatment protocols in dialogue with international experts, and working with health policy makers in regional and national institutions, Dr. Picon and colleagues are working hard to reverse some of the most pernicious effects of the pharmaceutical-ization of health care in their part of the world. These scientists and public health physicians seek to understand the effects of academic-industry relationships on the processes and outcomes of biomedical research. They do not reject the power of pharmaceuticals, but neither are they enamored of them. Their work is informed by a continued commitment to the scientific method, combined with a systemic critique of the political economy of pharmaceuticals as it plays out locally and a desire to empower public institutions to promote individual and collective rights to health. Like One-World Health's initiative, these scientists recombine elements that are available, taking the drugs and information that are already on hand, addressing their inherent limits, and maximizing their possibilities. They go a step further. As they work to scale their counterscience up through various political and legal channels, they challenge health policy makers in other middle- and low-income countries to deal with the avalanche of pharmaceutical globalization.

As these scientists engage the withdrawal and acquiescence of the state, particularly in the field of medical research and drug marketing, they are crafting a new public out of the public/private matrix that facilitates global experimentality. In their growing number of reference centers, they apply new protocols aimed at treatment continuity and comprehensive care—all the while striving to eliminate the "triage" that is implied in the current system of drug distribution. As these researchers gather patient data systematically, they also educate local judges to make sure that the clinical evidence they produce will have weight in the courts. Against institutional odds, they are creating their own brand of postmarketing surveillance for drugs that are widely used. The group takes into account the "real-life Brazilian patient" whose clinical and medical circumstances do not correspond to those of the "ideal" or highly edited subjects of clinical trials.

In politicizing the dominant role of pharmaceuticals in health-care policy, Dr. Picon and colleagues expose the organizational cultures that can compromise research integrity and safety, and they create the tools that make "a good science able to guide public health" possible. They are also making companies more accountable to the local contexts in which they run clinical trials. There is an element of contingency and surprise and motion here as notions of medical expertise are refined and as new institutional collaborations take form.

Such medical and institutional innovation is a critical facet of global health seen from the bottom up, revealing the potentially consequential role local scientists, academics, and policy makers can play. Illuminating these off-center and intricate practices and exploring their authoritative reach is a crucial task for public anthropology, especially in a time when political imagination is being largely tagged to market hopes and solutions or to top-down diplomacies. These alternative approaches reveal the plasticity that is built into the scientific experiment in its commercial and noncommercial forms and provide a way to bridge research and public health needs. In dissecting clinical trials and in redefining therapeutic value beyond their confines, these experimenters, along with many others yet to be heard, engender medical efficacy. They create alternative building blocks for the future of global medicine.

ACKNOWLEDGMENTS

Many people in the United States, Brazil, and Poland took the time to converse with me and to share their ideas, expertise, and experience. Dedicated professionals invited me into their worlds, opened a space of collective reflection, and made the issues discussed in this book relevant and palpable. Except in cases where individuals chose to be identified, I have maintained their anonymity to the extent possible by using pseudonyms and creating composite characters and entities that do not refer to any specific businesses. I am deeply grateful to them as well as to colleagues in Brazil for their long-term engagement and discussions with me. I especially thank Dr. Paulo Picon, a model of collaborative thinking and wit, as well as Dr. Andry Costa, Dr. Guilherme Sander, Indara Saccilotto, Patricia Picon, and many others, who have contributed greatly to this project. A number of clinicians have helped me to sort out ethical and technical dilemmas and through it all never lost sight of their role as caregivers. In Poland, I express my gratitude to Professor Zygmunt Sadovsky, Ewa Ksiezycka, Jolanta Zagrodzka, and Jerzy Szmagalski for their warm hospitality and orientation, as well as to the many clinicians and clinical trial investigators who provided me with insights into their work.

Over the years, I have learned in countless ways from the anthropological wisdom of Paul Rabinow, Michael Fischer, Ann Stoler, Veena Das, James Boon, Carol Greenhouse, and Rayna Rapp. Arthur Kleinman, to whom I am ever thankful, pushed me to think deeper about the dimensionality of the issues. Many scholars on different occasions provided important commentary and reflection. I thank Margaret Lock, Virginia Dominguez, Vincanne Adams, Philippe Bourgois, Marcia Inhorn, Nancy Scheper-Hughes, Jean Comaroff, John Comaroff, Didier Fassin, Allan Young, Deborah Gordon, Lawrence Cohen, Michael Lynch, Bruce Grant, Annelise Riles, Miriam Ticktin, Ilpo Helén, Ilana Feldman, Joseph Dumit, Kaushik Sunder Rajan, Deborah Poole, Mark Nichter, Allan Brandt, Rena Lederman, Helen Epstein, Joe Amon, Donald Light, Burton Singer, John Lantos, Aslihan Sanal, Natasha Schull, Susann Wilkinson, Clara Han, Mary Murrell, Andrew Lakoff, Joseph Harrington, Richard Cone, Peter Redfield, Ian Whitmarsh, Thomas Schlich,

Joseph Masco, and the late Iris Marion Young. Susan Reynolds Whyte and Michael Whyte engaged the ideas presented here during one memorable respite by the sea. I owe a very special debt to Harry Marks, whose comments on this project early on and subsequent reading of the manuscript were influential and invaluable.

I wrote a first version of this book while I was a member of the School of Social Science of the Institute for Advanced Study at Princeton in 2003–2004, and I am grateful for the support of the school's faculty, including Joan Scott, the late Clifford Geertz, Eric Maskin, Michael Waltzer, and fellows Carl Elliott, Tod Chambers, Trudo Lemmens, Joseph Davis, Leigh Turner, Charles Bosk, Raymond de Vries, Louis Charland, and Noam Zohar. I have benefited in myriad ways from exchanges with colleagues and students as I presented this work to the departments of anthropology at Princeton University, Harvard University, the University of Chicago, the University of Washington, the University of Michigan, and the Johns Hopkins University; as well as in the Department of the History of Science at Harvard University; the Program in Science, Technology, and Environmental Policy at Princeton; the Center for Bioethics and the Department of History and Sociology of Science at the University of Pennsylvania; the MacLean Center for Clinical Medical Ethics at the University of Chicago; the University of Toronto's Faculty of Law; McGill University's Department of Social Studies of Medicine; the Program in Medical Anthropology at the University of California, San Francisco; and the Program in Science, Technology, and Society at the Massachusetts Institute of Technology.

It has been a great pleasure to be part of the Department of Anthropology at the University of Pennsylvania. For their commitment to excellence and support, I thank all my colleagues, especially Greg Urban, Asif Agha, Brian Spooner, Jeremy Sabloff, Janet Monge, Kathy Hall, Sandra Barnes, John Jackson, Peggy Sanday, Fran Barg, Deborah Thomas, Claudia Valeggia, Paula Sabloff, Gautam Ghosh, Eduardo Fernandez-Duque, and Larysa Carr; as well as colleagues in the History and Sociology of Science, particularly Ruth Cowan, Susan Lindee, Robert Aronowitz, and Steven Feierman. I was also fortunate to have been part of the New School for Social Research where I benefited from dialogue with Jeffrey Goldfarb, Richard Bernstein, Benjamin Lee, Nancy Fraser, Jay Bernstein, Lawrence Hirschfeld, Arjun Appadurai, Vera Zolberg, Vijayanthi Rao, Hylton White, and Dan McIntyre. Students over the years have been an inspiration, giving the spark to move ideas along and offering new directions. I thank them all, and especially Karolina Szmagalska-Follis, Joanna Radin, Erica Dwyer, Hannah Voorhees,

Simanti Dasgupta, Grzegorz Sokol, and Imogen Bunting, who tragically passed away in 2006 as she entered her intellectual prime. Michael Joiner, Alex Gertner, and Ari Samsky read sections and versions and offered outstanding feedback. Thanks to Amy Saltzman, Steven Porter, and Matthew Goldberg for always constructive conversation; and Joyce Meng, David Laslett, and Brett Perlmutter, who provided stellar research assistance as well as the last needed push. I also thank Nicole Luce-Rizzo, Kathy Mooney, Ilana Porter, Charles Whitcroft, Márcia Sartori Colombo, Linda Forman, Isabel Teixeira, and Peg Hewitt for research support and/or crucial editorial feedback at various stages of the project.

This work was supported by the Crichton Fund (Department of Anthropology of Harvard University), the National Endowment for the Humanities, the Wenner-Gren Foundation Individual Research Grant, Richard Carley Hunt Fellowship; and the School of Social Science, Institute for Advanced Study, Princeton. Any conclusions, findings, or recommendations are my own and not necessarily those of sponsoring agencies. Chapter 1 contains revised material that was first published in "Ethical Variability: Drug Development and the Globalization of Clinical Trials," *American Ethnologist* 32(2) (May 2005): 183–197; and in "Clinical Trials Offshore: On Private Sector Science and Public Health," *BioSocieties* 2 (April 2007): 21–40.

Fred Appel has been a remarkable editor and supporter of this book, giving patient and always engaged editorial guidance at many junctures. I was extremely lucky and am grateful to be working again with Lauren Lepow, production editor, as well as with the talented Maria Lindenfeldar and Bob Bettendorf.

For their constancy, friendship, compassion, and care, I thank Robert and Lorna Kimball, Guilherme and Fernanda Streb, Oksana and Andriy Falenchuk, Peter Johnson, Peter Yi, Sarah Hirschman, Laura Jardim, Hilary Friedman, Alya Sen, Elsja Reiss, Melissa Walker, Cristina Netto, Carol Zanca, and Linda Mannheim. I am forever grateful to Noemia Biehl as well as to my wonderful parents, Michael Petryna and Tania Petryna, and Mark Petryna and Luba Veverka who have taught me so much.

My greatest debt is to my husband João Biehl, who helped me immensely in the thinking and writing of this book. We conducted interviews together in Brazil, and João drew from his deep knowledge of ethics and politics and of Brazil; no stone was left unturned. Thank you, João, for your care, generosity, and love. You and Andre are the joy of my life.

NOTES

⛥

Introduction

1. A protocol outlines a study's objectives, design, method, statistical approach, and organization.

2. See the seminal work *Strangers at the Bedside* (Rothman 1991).

3. Parexel's *Bio/Pharmaceutical R&D Statistical Sourcebook 2008/2009*, p. 18.

4. The United States spends 14 percent of its gross domestic product on health care (more than any other industrialized nation), and prescription costs are the fastest-growing component of the U.S. health-care market. Drug companies consistently spend more on lobbying than do other industries. Emerging markets constitute 17 percent of the global market, and they are outpacing traditional markets in terms of growth. They were expected to contribute 30 percent of the market's total growth in 2007 (http://open.imshealth.com/webshop2/IMSinclude/i_article_20061204a.asp).

5. These data derive from the "National Ambulatory Medical Care Survey 2005 Summary," Division of Health Care Statistics, Centers for Disease Control and Prevention. See Cherry, Woodwell, and Rechtsteiner 2005:5.

6. I focus on the use of trials as a source of treatment, not as a source of income. For the latter, see Abadie 2009; Elliott 2007; and Harkness 1996.

7. My focus is primarily on drugs, not vaccines or medical devices, and on noncommunicable rather than communicable diseases such as HIV/AIDS. Also, my study focuses primarily on industry-sponsored research, although I explore how public and private spheres of research overlap and document academic responses to the effects of industry-sponsored research in Brazil.

8. See Parexel 2005:35; CenterWatch 2005:162. Outsourced clinical development expenditures reportedly reached $23 billion in 2008, doubling from $11.2 billion in 2003. On CRO market size estimates, see http://www.acrohealth.org/industry-ataglance.php.

9. On the aftermath of the Chernobyl nuclear disaster, see Petryna 2002. On global pharmaceuticals, see Petryna, Lakoff, and Kleinman 2006.

10. See Healy 2006; Moynihan and Cassels 2005; Sackett and Oxman 2003, for example.

Chapter One: Ethical Variability

1. My interlocutors use the terms "patient" and "subject" interchangeably.

2. On informal networks of medicinal access and polytherapy, see Das and Das 2006. On the field of pharmaceutical anthropology as the analysis of the

contexts of medicines, "the constellations of cultural meanings and social rela-tions within which medicines exist in a given time and place," and the coexis-tence of Western and indigenous medicines, see van der Geest and Whyte 1988:3; also see van der Geest, Whyte, and Hardon 1996. Other pioneering works in the field include Kleinman 1981; Hardon 1987; Nichter and Vukovic 1994; Etkin 1999; Biehl 2005; and Lakoff 2006b.

3. Anthropologists and sociologists of science and medicine are devoting considerable attention to clinical research in a variety of global settings. See, for example, DelVecchio Good 2001; Adams 2003; Biehl 2007; Dumit forthcoming; Fisher 2009; Geissler and Molyneux (in press); Geissler et al. 2008; Konrad 2007; Kuo 2005; Nguyen 2005; Salter, Cooper, and Dickins 2006; Sunder Rajan 2005, 2006, 2007.

4. Clinical trials can begin only after trial sponsors have submitted an inves-tigational new drug (IND) application to the FDA. The IND application is reviewed by the FDA and a panel of scientists and nonscientists in hospitals and research institutions approves the research. Data derived from preclinical and clinical research and the analyses of how a drug behaves are submitted in the form of a new drug application, in which the drug sponsor asks the FDA to con-sider approving a new drug for marketing in the United States (http://www.fda .gov/fdac/features/2002/402_drug.html).

5. See Parexel 2008:2. Spending by the top ten biopharmaceutical compa-nies represents roughly 60 percent of total industry R&D spending.

6. For a critical examination of the FDA's adoption of this four-phase ap-proach, see Carpenter (in press).

7. For earlier concerns about the future of the clinical trials enterprise, see Meinert 1988.

8. Phase 4 studies are also significantly outsourced. The pharmaceutical in-dustry outsources not only research and development but also manufacturing, packaging, distribution, and sales and marketing activities.

9. Four hundred and sixty-two were operating in North America and Eu-rope alone in 2006 (CenterWatch 2008:227). On the industry dynamics of out-sourcing, see Rettig 2000 and Milne and Paquette 2004.

10. In 2006, of all clinical investigators who filed with the FDA (via a so-called 1572 form), 73.1 percent were from North America, 12.1 percent from Western Europe, 6.2 percent from Central-Eastern Europe, 4.1 percent from Asia-Pacific, 2.9 percent from South America, and 1.5 percent from the Middle East and Africa (Centerwatch 2008:455). Between 2001 and 2006, the annual growth in active investigators in these countries was as follows: India (48.6 per-cent), China (30.9 percent), Russia (28.8 percent), Argentina (21.6 percent), Brazil (16 percent), Costa Rica (12.9 percent), and Poland (8.4 percent). See Tufts CSDD Analysis of FDA's Bioresearch Monitoring Information System File (BMIS).

11. See Sim and Detmer 2005.

12. On clinical trials as negotiated social order, see Marks 1997:134.

13. For overviews and case studies of research abuses among minorities and other disadvantaged groups, see Reverby 2000; Jones 1981 [1993]; Lederer 1997;

Moreno 2000; and Rothman 1991, among others. For critiques of the U.S. system for developing, testing, and using prescription drugs, see Abramson 2004; Angell 2005; Goozner 2004; Avorn 2004; Kassirer 2004; Moynihan and Cassels 2005.

14. For discussion of the secrecy in pharmaceutical research, see Angell 2005. Also see Goozner 2004. On gag clauses, see Steinbrook 2005. On the need to register clinical trials, see Dickersin and Rennie 2003.

15. In an article entitled "Sponsorship, Authorship and Accountability," Frank Davidoff et al. write, "[C]orporate sponsors have been able to dictate the terms of participation in the trial, terms that are not always in the best interests of academic investigators, the study participants or the advancement of science generally. Investigators may have little or no input into trial design, no access to the raw data, and limited participation in data interpretation. These terms are draconian for self-respecting scientists, but many have accepted them because they know that if they do not, the sponsor will find someone else who will" (2001:1232–1233). On pharmaceutical industry sponsorship and research outcome and quality, see Lexchin et al. 2003. Also see Bodenheimer 2000. For the CRO industry's response to criticism, see Kuebler et al. 2002.

At the time I was conducting my research, the CRO industry organized ACRO (Association for Clinical Research Organizations). It is now the main lobbying and trade organization for the world's largest CROs. Medical journal articles critical of CROs have cited several cases involving CROs that have gone wrong, including the TeGenero monoclonal antibody study and the Adventis (now Sanofi-Adventis) trial for the antibiotic Ketek. In response to these criticisms, ACRO notes that the thousands of studies in which CROs act well within regulatory rules are ignored. In both cases, CROs were not held liable (Redfearn 2008).

16. I have aggregated the experiences of the researchers and businesspeople I spoke to into two companies. These company names are pseudonyms and do not refer to any actual business.

17. Lapses in monitoring or violations of integrity can cause data to be excluded. This, in turn, can raise questions about the validity of the results of the overall trial, which can be a "PR disaster or [can] kill a drug," as one pharmaceutical scientist told me.

18. In fact, Poland lost its lead in the clinical trials market that year. See "Annual Growth in Active Investigators by Select Countries," Tufts CSDD Analysis of FDA Bioresearch Monitoring Information System File (BMIS).

19. On benefit sharing as a mode of "giving back," see Hayden 2007. On the value added to the research enterprise by patients and subjects, see Merz et al. 2002.

20. Me-too drugs are considered less innovative because FDA approval of drugs is generally made on the basis of a drug's superiority to a placebo, not its superiority to existing drugs. FDA data show that 53 percent of the drugs approved between 1982 and 1991 offered "little or no therapeutic gain." Between 1996 and 2001, "[t]he pharmaceutical companies' spending on research and de-

velopment increased by 40 percent, but the number of new drugs reaching the market decreased by 50 percent. Of 31 'blockbuster' drugs . . . launched between 1992 and 2001, 23 were me-too drugs for common conditions such as allergies and inflammation" (Lansbury 2004: B02).

21. On payment to Phase 1 trial subjects, see Elliott 2008 and Abadie 2006. On the ethics of early-stage gene transfer trials, see Kimmelman 2007.

22. See also Parexel 2005:46.

23. Among the ten leading global pharmaceutical markets, the United States ranks first and holds a 60.5 percent share. Germany, France, Italy, the UK, Spain, and Belgium also rank among the top ten. Combined, they hold a 21 percent share, followed by Japan (15.1 percent), Canada (2.4 percent), and Australia (1.1 percent) (http://www.imshealth.com).

24. For further discussion on the "pill-taking life," see James Gorman's essay "The Altered Human Is Already Here" (2004). The author characterized this treatment saturation as a "kind of leap into the posthuman future. [The] jump is biochemical, mediated by proton-pump inhibitors, serotonin boosters and other drugs that have become permanent additives to many human bloodstreams. Over the past half-century, health-conscious, well-insured, educated people in the United States and in other wealthy countries have come to take being medicated for granted. More people shift to the pill-taking life every year, to the delight of pharmaceutical manufacturers."

25. Also see work by Lowy 2000; Hilts 2004; and Daemmrich 2004, among others. Minority groups continue to be underrepresented in certain health research, For example, in 1996, African American patients represented 11 percent of all cancer trial participants; by 2002 that number declined to 7.9 percent. Hispanics, who make up 9.1 percent of the U.S. population, made up only 3 percent of participants in clinical trials in 2002, down from 3.7 percent in 1996 (Murthy et al. 2004). However, Wendler et al. 2006 report "very small differences in the willingness of minorities, most of whom were African-Americans and Hispanics in the U.S., to participate in health research compared to non-Hispanic whites" (2006:0201).

26. See U.S. Department of Health and Human Services 1998:2005.

27. For earlier skepticism regarding the substantiality of subgroup differences, see Piantadosi and Wittes 1993 and Meinert 1995. For a different perspective on statistical issues, see Bailey 1994.

28. According to Parexel, "new clinical research starts soared 39% to a record high of 542 in 2004" (2005:49).

29. The out-migration of clinical research to so-called nontraditional research areas signals a change in a fundamental assumption in clinical trials participation. In the new clinical trials "markets," citizens are not the long-term beneficiaries of new drugs. The reciprocal cycle of test subjects typically conceived of as end users/consumers of drugs is being broken (Petryna 2005).

30. On the thalidomide scandal, see Stephens and Brynner 2001.

31. Testing requirements are typically established by national regulatory agencies, and they can differ from country to country; duplicate testing threat-

ened to delay foreign market access and affect the global trade in pharmaceuticals. Japan, perceived to be a potential large consumer market for U.S. pharmaceuticals, is famous for its intransigent regulatory system. See Applbaum 2006.

32. This estimate is given by the Association for Clinical Research Organizations (http://www.acrohealth.org/trends.php).

33. For an assessment of the commercialization of ethical review boards, see Lemmens and Freedman 2000.

34. As a result, investigators and trial monitors have to be more careful so as not to include patients who are too sick, or "ineligible patients. You may be providing treatment to someone who may not need it," as this scientist put it.

35. On trials as surrogates to health care in Uganda, see Reynolds Whyte et al. 2006.

36. For example, it was reported that "almost 1 of 10 US physicians currently engaged in a formal consultancy with the investment industry" (Topol and Blumenthal 2005:2654). Also see Brody 2007.

37. OIG 2001:12–13. FDA auditors ensure "the quality integrity of data submitted to FDA to demonstrate the safety and efficacy of regulated products, and to determine that human rights and the welfare of human and animal research subjects are adequately protected." Such oversight forms are indeed the successful product of public efforts to establish regulatory standards and legal mandates for the conduct of human biomedical research, particularly in vulnerable settings.

38. See the work of Benatar 2001; Benatar and Singer 2000; Farmer 2002; OIG 2001; Rothman 2000; Schuklenk and Ashcroft 2000.

39. On critiques of the ethics committee model, see Bosk 1999, 2002, 2005; Bosk and de Vries 2004; de Vries 2004; Guillemin 1998; Lederman 2006. On the deflection of attention from structural injustices, see Farmer 2003; Macklin 2004; Chambliss 1996; Marshall and Koenig 2004. Anthropological works on the ethics of biotechnology and new medical technologies have deepened the analysis of new biomedical technologies as they affect new patterns of civic, medical, and commercial organization (Biehl 2001; Cohen 1999; DelVecchio Good 2001; Dumit 2000; Franklin 1995; Lock 2001; Petryna 2002; Rapp 1999; Scheper-Hughes 2004; Strathern 1992). This body of work examines an important dimension of ethics beyond its universal and regulatory (or normative) frameworks. New technologies raise new contexts of decision making over doing what is right; thus, beyond defining instances of moral certainty, ethics also involves a set of tactics that can be generative of new human conditions and events (Fischer 2001, 2003; Rabinow 1996, 2003). For earlier warnings on the dangers of ethics' becoming disassociated from the empirical realities it claims to know, see Jonas 1969 and Toulmin 1987.

40. The United States should not be vaunted as the standard-bearer for adequate protection, and many problems of oversight that afflict human research in this country accompany the offshore trial.

41. I hope that it is obvious that I do not invoke variability as a sweeping generalization of the quality of ethical review in various countries.

42. For perspectives on this controversy, see Angell 1988, 1997, 2000; Bayer 1998; Botbol-Baum 2000; Crouch and Arras 1998; de Zulueta 2001; Lurie and Wolfe 1998, 2000; Rothman 2000.

43. The placebo-control trial typically consists of a placebo arm and a treatment arm. Its alternative, the active-control trial, consists of an arm of treatment with known efficacy (active control) and an experimental arm.

44. See the works of Jones 1981 [1993]; Brandt 1978; and Reverby 2000.

45. In support of this view, and in response to Angell's 1997 essay, in which her criticism of the use of placebo groups in randomized clinical trials appears, a group of scientists from developed and developing countries wrote: "Many would judge [inequalities in treatment access] to be offensive to our ethical systems that hold all human lives to be of equal value, but nonetheless the profound injustice in the global distribution of health resources is ugly but real.... If [Angell's critique] is accepted then the implications for medical research on the health problems of poor countries are profound. Many cheap interventions that have been shown to reduce mortality and morbidity in [poor countries] could never have been properly evaluated. Without valid data on effectiveness, it is unlikely that measures such as oral rehydration therapy, vitamin A supplementation, and syndromic treatment of sexually transmitted diseases would have been widely adopted, with the consequent loss of very many lives" (Aaby et al. 1997:1546).

46. Variability, however, is not meant to evoke the notion of "cultural relativism," although variability has been interpreted in such terms (Christakis 1992). Reliance on culture to explain differences in global health practices has been a central project in the field of medical anthropology for decades. Knowledge of such cultural differences, as translated into the health-care arena, tends to focus on "unbridgeable" moral divides between Western and non-Western groups. In the ethical imperialism versus relativism debate (Macklin 1999), anthropologists working in health-care arenas and elsewhere have been faulted for an alleged blind defense of local cultural tradition, making them susceptible to the "moral and intellectual consequences that are commonly supposed to flow from relativism—subjectivism, nihilism, incoherence, Machiavellianism, ethical idiocy, esthetic blindness, and so on" (Geertz 1984 [2000]:42). Medical anthropologists, by contrast, have recently contended that a focus on cultural and moral difference in health care can become dangerous to the very people and practices anthropologists have sought to understand, particularly in the contexts of massive epidemics and debates over treatment access. As Paul Farmer (1999) and Jim Yong Kim et al. (2003) and others point out, culture understood as difference has been used to explain "why" the poor are somehow less responsible regarding treatment regimes. Both Farmer and Kim have exposed the way moral assumptions in health planning can further entrench inequality, justifying some interventions while disallowing others. Their work and that of other anthropologists (Biehl 2007; Briggs and Mantini-Briggs 2003) moves beyond emphasis on difference and examines trajectories of local pandemics as they are influenced and remediated by international policy and choices.

47. See Petryna 2002; Smith 1990.

48. World Medical Association 2000:3044. This statement, of course, does not pertain to instances in which risk from withholding a proven therapy is lacking, as, for example, in the case of analgesics and antihistamines.

49. At stake in the placebo debate was more than the issue of standard of care and the global patients' right of access to it. The regulatory weight of the Helsinki declaration, the ability of IRBs to enforce proper research conduct globally, and the definition of just redistribution (particularly in resource-poor areas of the world) remained unaddressed.

50. For a description of how regulatory decisions can influence the definition of experimental groups, see Petryna 2005.

51. This is by no means an exhaustive review of this debate, which has been discussed and argued considerably, but a view into how ethical discourses are shaped by existing institutional interests.

52. In the context of HIV/AIDS care, sociologist Carol Heimer (2008) points to the confusion caregivers face in making distinctions between ethical norms and legal mandates, and rules that are meant as guidance and those meant to be followed exactly. Her important work points to the uneven landscape of implementation of international guidelines.

53. Negotiated in 1994, TRIPS is administered by the World Trade Organization (WTO) and sets minimum standards for many forms of intellectual property regulation within WTO member countries.

54. According to the Office of Inspector General, these are partial estimates. See OIG 2001. These numbers refer to New Drug Applications (NDAs) only, that is, applications made to the FDA to license and market drugs after they have been tested.

55. The Office of Inspector General stated that "among the countries that have experienced the largest growth in clinical investigators [for commercially sponsored trials] are Russia and countries in Eastern Europe and Latin America" (OIG 2001:i). Also see "Annual Growth in Active Investigators by Select Countries, Tufts CSDD Analysis of FDA's Bioresearch Monitoring Information System File (BMIS).

56. The OIG's mission statement is as follows: "The mission of the Office of Inspector General, as mandated by Public Law 95-452 (as amended), is to protect the integrity of Department of Health and Human Services (HHS) programs, as well as the health and welfare of the beneficiaries of those programs. The OIG has a responsibility to report both to the Secretary and to the Congress program and management problems and recommendations to correct them. The OIG's duties are carried out through a nationwide network of audits, investigations, inspections and other mission-related functions performed by OIG components." See Office of Inspector General at the Department of Health and Human Services (http://oig.hhs.gov/organization/OIGmission.html, downloaded September 2004).

57. The regulatory preference for the expansion of the IRB model was reflected in a National Bioethics Advisory Commission (2000) report recommending that studies submitted to the FDA receive ethical committee review

both in the United States and in the country in which research is being carried out (as opposed to the present situation, in which only foreign ethical review and approval are required). The report endorsed the idea of dual review with the provision that if host countries have working ethical review committees, then only approval of those committees is required.

58. I am grateful to Elaine Kusel for providing relevant legal documents.

59. Pfizer contracted a CRO, European based at the time, to organize the transfer of blood samples to its laboratory in Geneva to conduct assays on children's spinal fluid samples. The Trovan story illustrates how the political economy of drug development links seemingly disconnected worlds and jurisdictions. At the same time, the legal viability of existing international codes of human subjects protections is being thrown into doubt.

60. See Lewin 2001. On the politics of the 1996 cerebrospinal meningitis epidemic in Nigeria, see Ejembi, Renne, and Adamu 1998.

61. Pfizer was sued under the Alien Tort Claims Act (ATCA). In the case of Bhopal, for example, the ATCA was used to sue a transnational corporation for violating international law in a country outside the United States. "If these suits are allowed to proceed, then ATCA could become a powerful tool to increase corporate accountability." The Alien Tort Claims Act also "allows victims to sue human rights abusers in US courts, even if the infraction" occurred outside the United States. "Liability now seems to be expanding over time, distance, supply chains and incorporation, and with the growth of legal activism and a growing class-actions industry, particularly in North America, [corporate social responsibility] looks like [it is] turning into a risk management strategy" (http://www.globalpolicy.org/intljustice/atca/2005/0803morality.htm).

62. The Nuremberg Code was established as a response to Nazi medical experiments on prisoners in concentration camps. The code instituted norms of protection for subjects of scientific research experiments in the form of informed and voluntary consent and human rights guarantees.

63. In another instance of lawyers' attempting to eliminate ethical restrictions, rather than to assert them, see Alden 2004.

64. This expedient experimentality first caught my attention in the context of the scientific management of the Chernobyl nuclear crisis. See Petryna 2002.

65. The domain of international law in remunerating such violations requires careful assessment. This problematic has been outlined in Das's (1995) consideration of the Bhopal Union Carbide case.

66. Simon 2006; Topol 2004; Mathews and Martinez 2004; Psaty and Furberg 2005.

67. See Berenson 2007 on this point.

68. The recent multiple organ dysfunction and catastrophic immune response in six test subjects during an outsourced Phase 1 trial of the monoclonal antibody TGN1412 in England serves as an example.

69. On the commercialization and privatization of clinical research, see Mirowski and van Horn 2005; Fisher 2009.

70. There is currently a move to license sites just as you would a dentist's office, but the industry is avidly resisting this.

71. This point and the one about the economics of floater sites were made by participants in a conference on international clinical trials (November 2004), including a representative of a large CRO and the owner of a small U.S.-owned clinical trials company.

72. The quotation continues: "the inclusion of an independent endpoints committee should be the rule, and exceptions to this rule should be justified" (Juni et al. 2004:2025).

73. The idea that adversities stemming from the drug can be obscured by "normal" background risks in a given context was the argument the FDA used to explain why it failed to flag Vioxx as risky: "The national adverse event reporting system that helps the FDA flag dangerous side effects was of little use in this case because the ailments possibly caused by Vioxx—heart attacks and strokes—are so common" (Masters and Kaufman 2004:A01).

74. U.S. researchers have made much the same point regarding the use of new arrhythmia and other coronary disease "prevention" drugs. Even in the overrich United States, there is advocacy for more economic and more equitable treatments. On pharmaceutical trials and the marketing of chronic disease, see Greene 2006.

75. On the reverse engineering of standards, see Bowker and Star 1999.

Chapter Two: Arts of Drug Development

1. From Satire 5, Donne 2007:111.

2. On the politics of difference in medical research, see Epstein 2007; also see Lippman 2006 and Whitmarsh 2008. On the making of an "ethnic" drug, see Kahn 2004.

3. On the concept of pharmaceutical paternalism, see Fisher 2009. Also see Abadie 2009.

4. Gene therapy trials, for example, entail more technological complexity and planning, and costs per patient tend to be higher. Costs also vary according to type of recruitment advertising (involving letter writing, phone screening, or database mining). Other factors include the complexity of documentation in case report forms; institutional review board fees and costs of complying with regulations; trial insurance and compensation for serious adverse events (or SAEs). Each type of SAE typically has a cost of documentation attached to it; payments are made to study coordinators for filling out SAE forms and reporting them to institutional review boards and/or data and safety monitoring boards.

5. Dr. Besselaar passed away unexpectedly in 2004 at the age of seventy. http://www.towntopics.com/mar2404/obits.html.

6. Some of the information recounted here is also publicly available.

7. For detailed accounts of this case, see Stephens and Brynner 2001 and Daemmrich 2004.

8. According to Harry Marks, "That the FDA from the onset of the 1938 law sought to regulate claims of therapeutic benefit is clear, despite subsequent political and legal challenges from industry which forced the FDA to get specific

statutory authority to examine claims of drug efficacy" (2008:29n.5). Also see Marks 1997 and Daemmrich 2004.

9. "Randomization to treatment groups and double-blinding are two ways used to minimize bias in clinical trials. . . . Blinding is used in conjunction with randomization. Single-blinding means the participant doesn't know whether he or she is receiving the experimental product, an established treatment for that disease, or a placebo—but the research team does know what the participant is receiving. Clinical trials are usually double-blinded, meaning that neither the participant nor the research team knows during the trial which participants receive the experimental product." See http://www.fda.gov/fdac/features/2007/207_trials.html.

10. On the concept of regulatory science as a field of negotiation between scientists and policy makers, see Jasanoff 1998.

11. Similarly, University of Chicago economist Sam Peltzman analyzed the new drug amendments and argued that the cost of compliance with them would reduce drug innovation (1973). See Daemmrich 2004.

12. I am very grateful to Harry Marks for pointing me to these issues and, specifically, to "experimentality" at work at the outset of modern drug regulation, which he illustrates in his book *Progress of Experiment*.

13. On the Department of Health and Human Services' recent revisiting of the matter of prisoner research, see Lerner 2007.

14. On the complexity of historical actors involved in the following cases of research abuse, see Brandt 1978; Halpern 2001, 2004; Howell and Hayward 2003; Jones 1981 [1993]; Reverby 2000; Rothman and Rothman 2005. On the concept of "useful" bodies in twentieth-century medical experiments, see Goodman, McElligott, and Marks 2003.

15. It is very difficult to know how many died as a direct result of nontreatment. According to Jean Heller, "A 1969 study of 276 untreated syphilitics who participated in the Tuskegee study showed that 7 had died as a direct result of syphilis." Additional deaths could not be determined at that late date. "However, of the 400 men in the original syphilitic group, 154 died of heart disease . . . that was not specifically related to syphilis (2000:117). Tuskegee became a critical issue in the civil rights movement (Reverby 2000; Halpern 2001). "Radical social movements generalized the logic of civil rights to a range of other constituencies, including patients, institutionalized populations, and research subjects. In light of this new cultural ethos, risk-laden experiments acceptable during the preceding two decades could no longer be justified" (Halpern 2004:120).

16. Jonsen and Stryker 1993; Chadwick 1997.

17. *The Belmont Report* 1979.

18. This is based on Subpart C of 45 CFR 46 in the Code of Federal Regulations. The FDA had already established regulations concerning informed consent in the early sixties.

19. *The Belmont Report* 1979.

20. As stated in *The Belmont Report*, "An autonomous person is an individual capable of deliberation about personal goals and of acting under the direction of such deliberation. To respect autonomy is to give weight to autonomous persons'

considered opinions and choices while refraining from obstructing their actions unless they are clearly detrimental to others. To show lack of respect for an autonomous agent is to repudiate that person's considered judgments, to deny an individual the freedom to act on those considered judgments, or to withhold information neccessary to make a considered judgment, when there are no compelling reasons to do so."

21. There are, of course, other lineages of globalized research related to tropical medicine and colonial health services, experimentation in "island nations," and post–World War II international development in Africa, Asia, and Latin America. From Walter Reed's Yellow Fever Commission in Cuba to the experimental eradication of malaria in Cuba and Mauritius in the sixties to present AIDS and malarial vaccine research and clinical trials, most have involved government sponsorship and have often blurred lines between research experiment and provision of health services. See Packard 2007; Geissler et al. 2008; Whyte et. al. 2006, for example. On AIDS as a domain of expansion of transnational medicine, see Dodier 2005. Arguably, one of the first global trials linked to "population science" and with explicit industry ties began in 1956, when Searle, a British pharmaceutical company, launched worldwide trials for their oral contraceptive pill Enovid (Marks 2001). Initial field studies of the pill were carried out in Puerto Rico, believed to be well suited because it was outside the jurisdiction of the Comstock laws. These laws made the testing of contraceptives illegal in most U.S. states (ibid.:265). Moreover, it was an island with a stable population, excellent for monitoring research; and it hosted a large family-planning movement with networks of birthing clinics, excellent for attracting trial participants. As Lara Marks shows in her important book *Sexual Chemistry*, research on the oral contraceptive—the century's first "lifestyle" drug—combined charity and international development efforts with pharmaceutical market expansion. Similar public-private patterns and partnerships continue today in the context of AIDS (Biehl 2007).

22. With "dual use" drug testing, for example, it is much more difficult to trace the cause of adverse events. On psychopharmaceutical branding practices, see Healy 2006 and Greenslit 2005.

23. According to CenterWatch, outsourcing expenditure as a percentage of R&D expenditure increased as follows: 16.6 percent (2002); 19.2 percent (2004); 21.7 percent (2006); 24.7 percent (2008); 28.3 percent (projected for 2010) (2008: 262).

24. Jesse Gelsinger suffered multiple organ failure and brain death and died in the course of a gene therapy trial at the University of Pennsylvania in 1999. Ellen Roche died from lung and kidney failure during an asthma study at Johns Hopkins in 2001.

25. According to Pierre Azoulay (2003), an economist at MIT's Sloan School of Management, drug companies keep the more innovative research in-house, and CROs become "data-production sweatshops" for the more routinized and less innovative work of me-too Phase 3 trials (Azoulay cited in Shuchman 2007:1367).

26. In 1996, the burden of health-care cost containment moved signifi-

cantly from government toward third-party insurers. This shift yielded fewer reimbursements to physicians. The physician became his own agent of compensation, and clinical trials brought new opportunities for compensation. See Fisher (2009) for an incisive assessment of this dynamic.

27. Capitation in its harmful form is associated with reduction of services. "This is a service-reduction system in which individual providers may receive compensation for withholding services. Depending on patient needs for services, the financial risk in this new capitation scheme is shifted away from the insurance company or government entity and onto the doctor" (http://www .cascadepolicy.org/comments/capitate.htm, downloaded April 2004).

28. This cost was put at a much-contested $802 million in 2003. See DiMasi, Hansen, and Grabowski 2003. For a critique of this estimate and its methodological underpinnings, see Light and Warburton 2005.

29. The growth in the number of complaints against investigators grew as follows: 9 in 1998; 106 in 1999; 119 in 2000; 111 in 2001; 110 in 2002; 139 in 2003; 214 in 2004; 266 in 2005. It is unclear whether this increase is also an artifact of higher scrutiny.

30. "Trials of War Criminals" 1949.

31. For an analysis of the hazards of the research imperative, see Callahan 2003.

32. On the history and theory of informed consent, see Faden, Beauchamp, and King 1986.

33. On the limitations of vulnerability as a protection for human research participants, see Levine et al. 2004.

34. The 2000 Merck-sponsored study comparing the safety and efficacy of rofecoxib and over-the-counter naproxen in rheumatoid arthritis patients (Bombardier et al. 2000) aimed to show that rofecoxib did not damage the stomach as naproxen can. The VIGOR study, to be further detailed in the text, found that rofecoxib had the same effect as naproxen in terms of pain relief, and the rofecoxib group experienced only half the risk of gastrointestinal complications compared with naproxen. But it also showed a *fivefold* increase in the incidence of myocardial infarction (MI) in rofecoxib patients as compared with naproxen patients (Juni et al. 2004:2021). Merck spokesmen famously tried to explain away the finding by claiming that naproxen exhibited a "cardio protective" effect and that the difference in MI incidence is due primarily to this effect.

35. The chance that the drug could elevate cardiovascular risk "was raised in the medical review before Vioxx was approved" (Gilhooley 2007:946, cited from Psaty 2004).

36. According to current FDA regulation (21 CFR 213.52), "A sponsor may transfer responsibility for any or all of the obligations . . . to a contract research organization." Under such conditions, "A contract research organization that assumes any obligation of a sponsor shall comply with the specific regulations . . . applicable to this obligation and shall be subject to the same regulatory action as a sponsor for failure to comply with any obligation assumed under these regulations. Thus, all references to 'sponsor' . . . apply to a contract research organization to the extent that it assumes one or more obligations of the sponsor." See

http://www.accessdata.fda.gov/scripts/cdrh/cfdocs/cfCFR/CFRSearch.cfm?fr=312.52.

37. Dr. Steven Hirschfeld, quoted in Meadows 2002.

38. Pharmacogenomics, the study of how genes affect individual responses to drugs, for example, is said to potentially make drugs safer and less likely to produce adverse events by creating individualized genetic (or pharmacogenomic) profiles. If susceptibility to adverse drug reactions can be profiled, treatment—ideally—can be individually tailored to avoid such reactions.

39. U.S. Food and Drug Administration 2007.

Chapter Three: The Global Clinical Trial

1. Milosz 2004:25.

2. Their policy went into effect in July 2005.

3. World Health Organization International Clinical Trials Registry Platform, http://www.who.int/ictrp/en/, downloaded March 2007.

4. The estimate of fifty thousand includes commercial and noncommercial drug trials but excludes those involving medical devices and nonmedicinal interventions such as behavioral testing. Phase 4 postmarketing studies are also excluded. Also see CenterWatch 2005:91.

5. The average length of the phases of trials areas follows: one year for Phase 1, one and a half years for Phase 2, and three years for Phase 3.

6. CenterWatch 2005:16, 131.

7. The 2006 Phase 1 trial of the monoclonal antibody TGN1412 in Britain, which led to multiple organ dysfunction and catastrophic immune response in six test subjects, confirmed the nonnegotiable need for the registration of early trials. See Godlee 2006.

8. The mandate concerned intervention trials using drugs only. See *Guidance for Industry* 2002. Other significant registries are the European Clinical Trials Database (EudraCT) and the UK-based International Standard Randomised Controlled Trial Number Register. The main purpose of ClinicalTrials.gov is to facilitate patient access to clinical research. By contrast, EudraCT, launched in 2005, does not make such data publicly available. Although it allows national monitors to gather data on trial-related, unexpected serious adverse reactions, the rationale for the database is more administrative than clinical. It facilitates communications among national regulatory agencies over the content, commencement, and termination of trials in the European Union.

9. International Federation of Pharmaceutical Manufacturers & Associates. International Clinical Trials Registry Platform (ICTRP): IFPMA comments to ICTRP consultation on delayed disclosure, 2006 (http://www.who.int/entity/ictrp/3005_IFPMA_25Jan06.pdf).

10. Estimates, particularly those developed by DiMasi, Hansen, and Grabowski (2003), are widely cited to justify national and international pricing policy. These estimates, according to one critic, "rationalize the blockbuster business model and obfuscate development of a better one" (Light 2008:327).

11. Invitation for Open Comments, Pfizer response, January 2006: 6 (http://www.who.int/ictrp/consultation/en/index.html).

12. Ibid.

13. See "Comments on Disclosure Timing, Submission to WHO International Clinical Trials Registry Platform," January 2006:1 (http://www.who.int/ictrp/3009_Michael_Goodyear_Lisa_Golec_25Jan06.pdf).

14. http://www.who.int/ictrp/consultation/en/index.html, downloaded March 2007.

15. PricewaterhouseCoopers 2006.

16. "Apart from the effective transfer of the capital associated with the global trials conducted at home, the [$322 million] also comprises reduced expenditure for the purchase of medicines in hospital budgets. Pricewaterhouse-Coopers 2006:2.

17. For incisive critiques and reflections on these developments globally, see Stiglitz 2002; Sachs 2006; Klein 2007.

18. On postsocialist labor politics and on how vast numbers of workers without jobs got silenced in this transition, see Ost 2005.

19. http://www.warsawvoice.pl/view/11657, downloaded March 2007.

20. PricewaterhouseCoopers 2006:1.

21. See Petryna 2002 and Rivkin-Fish 2005, for example.

22. In addition to these frontier dynamics, anthropologists have shown how entrepreneurs and local governments deploy international rules and conventions as a mode of governance and to achieve ends other than those originally intended. On organ trafficking, see Scheper-Hughes 2004; on criminal violence in the postcolony, see Comaroff and Comaroff 2006; on unsanctioned wealth and economic regulation, see Roitman 2004.

23. "As defined by article 2 and article 19 of EU Clinical Trial Directive 2001/20/EC), the sponsor can be an individual, a company, an institution or an organisation. The sponsor does not need to be located in an EU Member State but has to have a legal representative in the EU" (http://www.ct-toolkit.ac.uk/_db/_documents/ClinicalTrialQ&A_24-01-05.pdf, downloaded April 2007).

24. *Applied Clinical Trials*, December 2002, 25, "Clinical Trials Terminology," Actmagazine.com, downloaded March 2007.

25. Compassionate use refers to a trial sponsor's providing a drug to a patient on charitable grounds. In open label extension (OLE) studies, patients who were assigned to treatment in the primary study are reassigned to active therapy to evaluate long-term safety issues. Both take place while an experimental therapy awaits final regulatory approval. There are significant concerns with OLE studies. "[I]ndividual participants may be invited to participate in the OLE without knowing their treatment status in the primary study (e.g. active drug or placebo), and before aggregate data about efficacy and safety have been analyzed. This means that subjects previously doing well on placebo or low doses of the drug will be enrolled in the OLE on active medication and often at a higher dose than they were taking previously" (http://www.uwo.ca/research/ethics/med/2g014-guideline-open-label-extension-studies-sep-1999.pdf, downloaded November 9, 2007).

26. There are several excellent English sources on the Warsaw ghetto and wartime history. See, for example, Krall 1996; Ringelblum 1974; Davies 2005.

27. A politician of the conservative party Prawo i Sprawiedliwość, Lech Kaczyński was inaugurated as president of Poland in 2005.

28. On insecurity in Poland, see Ost 2005. On economic exclusion and inclusion in Poland, see Pine and Haukanes 2005. Also see Wedel 1992; and on Poland beyond communism, see Nagengast, Buchowski, and Conte 2001.

29. This agency is called the Office for the Registration of Medicinal Products, Medical Devices and Biocidal Products. New clinical trials are registered in the Central Registry of Clinical Trials Unit.

30. This is not a pseudonym.

31. PricewaterhouseCoopers 2006:2.

32. Door-to-needle time denotes the time it takes to deliver a clot-busting medication to a heart failure patient entering an emergency room. It is a measure of excellence in cardiac care.

33. For an analysis of ethical issues in obtaining consent in emergency research, specifically in the context of thrombolytic drug development, see Brody 1995.

34. While much is known about how competitive wars over blockbuster market segments were waged, less is known about how these wars influenced clinical trials offshoring practices.

35. Companies were required by law to register their trials with state regulatory authorities and regionally based ethical review boards. Poland's six regional Chambers of Physicians would now house their own ethical review boards overseeing nonacademic research throughout Poland. On delays in implementation of law related to clinical research, see "Clinical Trials and Protection" 2007.

36. See Klein 1980 for an excellent review of Hirschman's ideas in the context of a competitive health-care market.

37. This tailoring of environment reflects, in Paul Rabinow's terms, assemblages, or a "distinctive type of experimental matrix of heterogenous elements, techniques, and concepts... They are comparatively effervescent, disappearing in years or decades, rather than centuries. Consequently, the temporality of assemblages is qualitatively different from that of either problematizations or apparatuses" (2003: 56). See also Ong and Collier 2005.

38. See Barry and Slater 2005.

39. See Ecks 2005; Biehl 2007; Dumit forthcoming.

40. For illuminating analyses of the concept of coercion and "misidentified" ethical concerns in the context of clinical research, see Hawkins and Emmanuel 2005 and Brody 2002. For a broad overview, see Wertheimer 2006.

41. Swedish Public Service Radio, Kalle Nilsson, "Astra Zeneca hotar med neddragningar," tisdag 20 juli 2004 (http://www.sr.se/ekot/artikel.asp?artikel=445969, downloaded July 27, 2004).

42. I am grateful to Joe Harrington for his insightful comments on "The Human Subjects Research Industry," a paper I presented at the Johns Hopkins Anthropology department in 2004.

43. In his book *Global "Body Shopping,"* anthropologist Xiang Biao explores

America's information technology (IT) industry and the India-based global labor management practice known as "body shopping." He argues that the outsourcing of IT services is so successful because of its local informal basis. Here, too, the mobility of industry is productive because it is able to free itself from state regulation of migration in this case (2006).

44. http://www.imshealth.com/ims/portal/front/articleC/0,2777,6599_3665_82713022,00.html, downloaded January 2008.

Chapter Four: The Aftermath of Clinical Trials

1. On the value structure of transnational pharmaceutical production, see Lakoff 2006a.

2. See Oxford Center for Evidence-Based Medicine, http://www.cebm.net/.

3. João Biehl and I met with this group annually from 2003 to 2006 to discuss medical research and the right to health in Brazil.

4. See *Jornal Gaucher*, no. 4 (April 2004): 1.

5. In other countries with comparable levels of development, the difference is only ten times greater, according to the Pan American Health Organization, http://www.paho.org.

6. Also see Mansfield 2006:09 and http://ramoslink.info/. On how companies subvert measures that would promote a more rational drug use policy, see Medawar and Hardon 2004.

7. On these disparities and their social consequences, see Scheper-Hughes 1992 and Biehl 2005.

8. On how efforts to solve social problems are less valued and replaced by the workings of the pharmaceutical "magic bullet," see Brandt 1985. On how definitions of treatable illness expand to enlarge drug markets and how sickness is sold, see Moynihan, Heath, and Henry 2002; Lexchin 2001; Healy 2006.

9. On the cost-effectiveness of treating the poor, see Farmer 2003.

10. The drug alglucerase was initially listed with the program. In 1998, imiglucerase was listed as a substitution for alglucerase.

11. Constituição do Brasil—Seção II—Da Saúde—Artigo 196.

12. In per capita terms, today public health spending is estimated at US$158 and private expenditure at US$225 per year (Pan American Health Organization). The broadening of health coverage did not go unnoticed by the pharmaceutical industry. The government would become a significant market, left as it was to provide high-cost procedures that private health plans chose not to cover (Elias and Cohn 2003).

13. Galvão 2002; Biehl 2007; Okie 2006; Dourada et al. 2006.

14. The guidelines focus on these and other conditions and diseases: acne, acromegalia, anemia, rheumatoid arthritis, asthma, dislipidemias, dystonias, Alzheimer's disease, Crohn's disease, Gaucher disease, Parkinson's disease, Wilson's disease, sickle cell disease, refractory epilepsy, Alexander disease, relapsing remitting muscular sclerosis, phenylketonuria, cystic fibrosis, chronic viral hepatitis B, chronic viral hepatitis C, congenital adrenal hyperplasia, congenital

hypothyroidism, neutropenia, osteoporosis, retreatment for chronic viral hepatitis B, ulcerative colitis, and renal transplantation.

15. http://www.fda.gov/orphan/progovw.htm, downloaded March 2007.

16. For a discussion of this drug in the context of the manufacturer's corporate citizenship campaigns, see Ecks 2008.

17. "Brand of the Year" 2004.

18. See Mansfield 2006.

19. This is a quotation from the municipal secretary of health in Goiânia, Otaliba Libânio. Mansfield 2006.

20. "Seminário discute ações judiciais sobre medicamentos excepcionais," http://www.agenciaminas.mg.gov.br/detalhe_noticia.php?cod_noticia=5812.

21. Cited from an interview with Dr. Paulo Picon. Mansfield 2006.

22. The disease belongs to a class of inherited disorders known as lysosomal storage disorders with incidences ranging from 1 in 40,000 to 1 in 200,000. This class includes forty rare disorders linked to an inherited enzyme deficiency. Gaucher disease is the nonneuronopathic adult form of the disease that is particularly common among Ashkenazi Jews, among whom the incidence is reported to be as high as 1 in 850. Roughly 35,000 to 40,000 people worldwide have been diagnosed with Gaucher disease. Only 3,000 patients are receiving enzyme replacement therapy, and this means fewer than 10 percent of sufferers are benefiting from treatment (http://www.gaucher.org.uk/furthermarch2002.htm).

23. The gene for the deficient enzyme was identified in 1981, and NIH researchers cloned it in 1984. The FDA granted U.S. marketing approval for Ceredase, an early version of enzyme replacement therapy, in 1991. Until that time, treatment for Gaucher mainly consisted of palliative measures. The focus here is on imiglucerase, which remains the standard of care. However, a new drug, miglustat, has recently been approved in the United States and Western Europe for the treatment of Gaucher. Other enzymes are also being tested for the treatment of the disease.

24. Fourteen years after the first version came to market, the maker can charge this price "because it can. There is no competition, patients are desperate and most insurers pay." See Anand 2005. The treatment remains out of reach for many patients in developing countries, and heated debates over its high cost continue as coalitions of patient groups battle the "access crisis" in the United States, the United Kingdom, and elsewhere (http://www.rarediseases.org/). The total global market of the enzyme replacement therapy is estimated to exceed US$1 billion (http://www.innkap.se/Press-Release).

25. Beutler noted that the "development of enzyme replacement therapy for Gaucher disease . . . is a triumph of translational medicine. At the same time, powerful commercial interests may have been influential in physicians adopting a high-dose rather than a low-dose treatment schedule. Moreover, the high cost of enzyme replacement therapy forces us to consider what society can afford" for very rare diseases (2004:118).

26. Andrew Pollack notes, "The standard Cerezyme [imiglucerase] dose—an infusion of 60 units of the drug per kilogram of body weight every two weeks—

was set in a clinical trial involving only 12 patients. Based on that trial, Ceredase, a nearly identical predecessor drug, was approved in 1991. Cerezyme, the same enzyme made differently, replaced it starting in 1994" (2008:A24).

27. See the opinion of Dr. Elisa Sobreira, a pediatrician in São Paulo. *Jornal Gaucher*, no. 3 (December 2003): 1–2.

28. I draw an analogy here with Bruno Latour's analysis of how French microbiologist Louis Pasteur "brought" anthrax into the laboratory and how, through the laboratory, he reformed French public health (1998).

29. The choice of outcome is typically made between a surrogate endpoint, a biological measurement, and a clinical ("hard") endpoint, such as death or pain relief. The latter is considered to represent evidence-based medicine, the former, a move away from it.

30. In Brazil as elsewhere it is common for doctors to juggle many positions in order to make it academically and financially.

31. On critiques of the exportation, marketing, and lax regulation of the distribution and sale of pharmaceuticals, see Melrose 1982; Silverman, Lee, and Lydecker 1982; Hardon 1987; Van der Geest and Whyte 1988; Van der Geest, Whyte, and Hardon 1996. Also see Scheper-Hughes 1992.

32. On the troubling history of statin promotion and the rise of "subjectively healthy but highly medicated" individuals in the United States, see Greene 2006.

33. Cited from "Notícias do CONASS," a journal of the Brazilian National Council for State Health Secretariats, June 20, 2007, http://www.conass.org, downloaded July 7, 2007.

34. See Renée Fox's classic rendering of experimental peril in a hospital ward, and how patients and physicians cope with uncertainty (1959).

35. The Brazilian clinical trials approval system is multilayered: a protocol must receive three sets of approvals before a clinical trial can be launched. It is initially approved by a local IRB, then CONEP, and then ANVISA.

36. "Uso de cobaias humanas" 2006.

37. See "Fiocruz culpa tradução."

38. "Uso de cobaias humanas" 2006.

39. *Jornal Gaucher*, no. 3 (December 2003): 2.

40. On how the capitalization of markets coincides with legal and regulatory norms and can create a set of safety compromises, see Jain 2006.

41. On the biotechnical embrace, see DelVecchio Good 2001.

Conclusion: The Future of Global Medicine

1. There is a parallel here with tobacco control as a public health strategy. See Gostin 2007.

2. See the review by Sami Timimi (2007) of a book I coedited entitled *Global Pharmaceuticals: Ethics, Markets, Practices* (2006).

3. See, for example, the work of Farmer 2003 and Pogge 2006.

4. See, for example, Frost, Reich, and Fujisaki 2002; Samsky 2008. For an indepth discussion of public-private partnerships, see Reich 2002; Moran 2005.

5. See PEPFAR 2006:107.

6. See the works and commentaries of Epstein 2007; Ramiah and Reich 2005; Halperin 2008; and Biehl 2007, for example.

7. Annelise Riles first identified this process of value reconciliation in the context of transnational institutional practices linked to women's rights (2005, 2004); see also Redfield 2006 for considerations of how this process occurs in global humanitarianism.

8. On international organizations and existing and unequal power relations between countries, see Garrett 2007; on efforts to politicize health seeking among the poorest, see Bannerjee, Deaton, and Duflo 2004.

9. See DNDWG 2001. Also see GFHR 2004.

10. Also see James Love, "Health Care and Intellectual Property: The Orphan Drug Act," http://ww.cptech.org/ip/healthorphan.

11. See http://www.oneworldhealth.org/.

12. *PIH Guide* 2006.

13. For a comparative analysis of pharmaceutical corporate social responsibility initiatives, see Meng 2007.

14. Dr. Paulo Picon, personal communication, 2006.

REFERENCES

Aaby, Peter, et al. 1997. "Ethics of HIV Trials." *Lancet* 350(9090):1546.

Abadie, Roberto. 2009. *A Guinea Pig's Wage: Risk, Body Commodifications, and the Ethics of Pharmaceutical Research in America.* Durham, NC: Duke University Press.

Abbasi, Kamran. 2005. "Developing European Clinical Research in the Interest of Patients and Public Health." PowerPoint presentation, Brussels.

Abraham, John. 2007. "Drug Trials and Evidence Bases in International Regulatory Context." *Biosocieties* 2:41–57.

Abramson, John. 2004. *Overdo$ed America: The Broken Promise of American Medicine.* New York: Harper Perennial.

ACHRE [Advisory Committee on Human Radiation Experiments]. 1996. "Final Report of the Advisory Committee on Human Radiation Experiments." Washington, DC: U.S. Government Printing Office.

Adams, Vincanne. 2003. "Randomized Controlled Crime: Postcolonial Sciences in Alternative Medicine Research." *Social Studies of Science* 32(5–6):659–690.

Alden, Edward. 2004. "US Interrogation Debate: Dismay at Attempt to Find Legal Justification for Torture." *Financial Times*, June 10, 3.

Amaral, K. M., J. G. Reis, and P. D. Picon. 2000. "Atenção Farmacêutica no Sistema Único de Saúde: Um Exemplo de Experiência bem Sucedida com Patientes Portadores de Hepatite C." *Revista Brasileira de Farmácia* 87:19–21.

Anand, Geeta. 2005. "Why Genzyme Can Charge So Much for Cerezyme." *Wall Street Journal*, November 16, A15.

Anderson, Warwick. 2003. *The Cultivation of Whiteness: Science, Health, and Racial Destiny in Australia.* New York: Basic Books.

Angell, Marcia. 1988. "Ethical Imperialism? Ethics in International Collaborative Clinical Research." *New England Journal of Medicine* 319(16):1081–1083.

———. 1997. "The Ethics of Clinical Research in the Third World." *New England Journal of Medicine* 337(12):847–849.

———. 2000. "Investigators' Responsibilities for Human Subjects in Developing Countries." *New England Journal of Medicine* 342(13):967–968.

———. 2004. "The Truth about the Drug Companies." *New York Review of Books* 51(12). Available at http://www.nybooks.com/articles/17244.

———. 2005. *The Truth about the Drug Companies: How They Deceive Us and What to Do about It.* New York: Random House.

———. 2006. "Your Dangerous Drugstore." *New York Review of Books* 53(10). Retrieved February 2007, from http://www.nybooks.com/articles/19055.

Annas, G. L., L. H. Glantz, and B. F. Katz. 1977. *Informed Consent to Human Experimentation: The Subject's Dilemma.* Cambridge, MA: Ballinger.

Applbaum, Kalman. 2006. "American Pharmaceutical Companies and the Adoption of SSRI's in Japan." In *Global Pharmaceuticals: Ethics, Markets, Practices,* edited by Adriana Petryna, Andrew Lakoff, and Arthur Kleinman, 85–111. Durham, NC: Duke University Press.

"Arexis AB: Arexis obtains orphan drug designation in the EU for novel cystic fibrosis therapy." 2005. Press Release. *Innovations Kapital.* Retrieved from http://www.innkap.se/PressRelease.aspx?page=5&press=173.

Arnold, David. 1993. *Colonizing the Body: State Medicine and Epidemic Disease in Nineteenth-Century India.* Berkeley and Los Angeles: University of California Press.

Austin, James, Diana Barrett, A. G. Breitenstein, Kent Buse, Laura Frost, Tomoko Fujisaki, Adetokunbo Lucas, Sheila McCarthy, William Muraskin, Clement Roberts, Marc Roberts, and Gill Walt. 2002. *Public-Private Partnerships for Public Health.* Edited by Michael R. Reich. Harvard Center for Population and Development Studies.

Avorn, Jerry. 2004. *Powerful Medicines: The Benefits, Risks, and Costs of Prescription Drugs.* New York: Knopf.

Azoulay, Pierre. 2003. "Agents of Embeddedness." NBER working paper 10142. December 2003. Cambridge, MA: National Bureau of Economic Research. Available at http://www.nber.org/papers/w10142.

Bailey, Kent. 1994. "Generalizing the Results of Randomized Clinical Trials." *Controlled Clinical Trials* 15:15–23.

Bannerjee, Abhijit, Angus Deaton, and Esther Duflo. 2004. "Wealth, Health, and Health Services in Rural Rajasthan." Poverty Action Lab Paper No. 8. Available at http://www.povertyactionlab.com.

Barnes, Kirsty. 2007. "PharmaNet to suffer formal SEC scrutiny." DrugResearcher .com. March 21, 2007. http://www.drugresearcher.com/news/, downloaded December 2007.

Barry, Andrew. 2001. *Political Machines: Governing a Technological Society.* London and New York: Athlone Press.

Barry, Andrew, and Don Slater, eds. 2005. *The Technological Economy.* London and New York: Routledge.

Bayer, R. 1998. "The Debate over Maternal-Fetal HIV Transmission Prevention Trials in Africa, Asia, and Caribbean: Racist Exploitation or Exploitation of Racism?" *American Journal of Public Health* 88(4):567–570.

The Belmont Report: Ethical Principles and Guidelines for the Protection of Human Subjects of Research. 1979. The National Commission for the Protection of Human Subjects of Biomedical and Behavioral Research. Washington, DC: Department of Health, Education and Welfare.

Benatar, Solomon. 2001. "Distributive Justice and Clinical Trials in the Third World." *Theoretical Medicine and Bioethics* 22(3):169–176.

Benatar, Solomon, and Peter A. Singer. 2000. "A New Look at International Research Ethics." *British Medical Journal* 321(7264):824–826.

Berenson, Alex. 2007. "Plaintiffs Find Payday Elusive in Vioxx Cases." *New York Times,* August 21, A1, A17.

———. 2008. "Study Reveals Doubt on Drug for Cholesterol." *New York Times*, January 15, A1, A16.

Beutler, Ernest. 1994. "Economic Malpractice in the Treatment of Gaucher's Disease." *American Journal of Medicine* 97(1):1–2.

———. 2004. "Enzyme Replacement in Gaucher Disease." *PLoS Medicine* 1(2): 118–121.

Biao, Xiang. 2006. *Global "Body Shopping": An Indian Labor System in the Information Technology Industry.* Princeton: Princeton University Press.

Biehl, João. 2001. "Technology and Affect: HIV/AIDS Testing in Brazil." *Culture, Medicine and Psychiatry* 25(1):87–129.

———. 2005. *Vita: Life in a Zone of Social Abandonment.* Berkeley and Los Angeles: University of California Press.

———. 2006. "Pharmaceutical Governance." In *Global Pharmaceuticals: Ethics, Markets, Practices*, edited by Adriana Petryna, Andrew Lakoff, and Arthur Kleinman, 206–240. Durham, NC: Duke University Press.

———. 2007. *Will to Live: AIDS Therapies and the Politics of Survival.* Princeton: Princeton University Press.

Bodenheimer, Thomas. 2000. "Uneasy Alliance—Clinical Investigators and the Pharmaceutical Industry." *New England Journal of Medicine* 342(20):1539–1544.

Bombardier, C., L. Laine, A. Reicin, et al. 2000. "Comparison of Upper Gastrointestinal Toxicity of Rofecoxib and Naproxen in Patients with Rheumatoid Arthritis." *New England Journal of Medicine* 343:1520–1528.

Bosk, Charles. 1999. "Professional Ethicist Available: Logical, Secular, Friendly. Bioethics and Beyond." *Daedalus* 128(4):47–68.

———. 2002. "Now That We Have the Data, What Was the Question?" *American Journal of Bioethics* 2(4):21–23.

———. 2005. *What Would You Do? The Collision of Ethnography and Ethics.* Chicago: University of Chicago Press.

———. 2007. "The New Bureaucracies of Virtue or When Form Fails to Follow Function." *PoLAR: Political and Legal Anthropology Review* 30(2):192–209.

Bosk, Charles, and Raymond de Vries. 2004. "Bureaucracies of Mass Deception: Institutional Review Boards and the Ethics of Ethnographic Research." *Annals of the American Academy of Political and Social Science* 595(1):249–263.

Botbol-Baum, Mylene. 2000. "The Shrinking of Human Rights: The Controversial Revision of the Helsinki Declaration." *HIV Medicine* 1(4):238–245.

Bowker, Geoffrey C., and Susan Leigh Star. 1999. *Sorting Things Out: Classification and Its Consequences.* Cambridge, MA: MIT Press.

Brada, Betsey. 2004. "Bodies of Evidence: The Emergence of AIDS Clinical Trials Group (ACTG) 076." *Newsletter of the AIDS and Anthropology Research Group* 16(2):7–8.

"Brand of the Year —Gleevec." 2004. *Med Ad News* 23(5):5.

Brandt, Allan M. 1978. "Racism and Research: The Case of the Tuskegee Syphilis Study." *Hastings Center Report* 8(6):21–29.

———. 1985. *No Magic Bullet A Social History of Venereal Disease in the United States since 1880.* New York: Oxford University Press.

Briggs, Charles, and Clara Mantini-Briggs. 2003. *Stories in the Time of Cholera: Racial Profiling during a Medical Nightmare.* Berkeley and Los Angeles: University of California Press.

Brody, Baruch. 1995. *Ethical Issues in Drug Testing, Approval, and Pricing: The Clot-Dissolving Drugs.* New York: Oxford University Press.

———. 2002. "Ethical Issues in Clinical Trials in Developing Countries." *Statistics in Medicine* 21:2853–2858.

Brody, Howard. 2007. *Hooked: Ethics, the Medical Profession, and the Pharmaceutical Industry.* Lanham, MD: Rowman & Littlefield.

Buekens, Pierre, Gerald Keusch, Jose Belizan, and Zulfiqar Ahmed Bhutta. 2004. "Evidence-Based Global Health." *Journal of the American Medical Association* 291(21):2639–2641.

Callahan, Daniel. 2003. *What Price Better Health? Hazards of the Research Imperative.* Berkeley and Los Angeles: University of California Press.

Canavan, Neil. 2008. "The Trouble with Trials." *Drug Discovery & Development,* March 1.

Canguilhem, Georges. 1991. *The Normal and the Pathological.* New York: Zone Books.

Caplan, Arthur. "Commentary: Report Paints Grim Picture of Drug Trial Safety." September 28, 2007. http://www.msnbc.msn.com/id/21029879/, downloaded October 5, 2007.

Carpenter, Dan. In press. *Reputation and Power: Organizational Image and Pharmaceutical Regulation at the FDA.*

CenterWatch. 2005. *State of the Clinical Trials Industry: A Sourcebook of Charts and Statistics.* Boston: Thomson CenterWatch.

———. 2007. "Glossary." Retrieved from http://www.centerwatch.com/patient/glossary.html#N.

———. 2008. *State of the Clinical Trials Industry: A Sourcebook of Charts and Statistics.* Boston: Thomson CenterWatch.

"CenterWatch Launches First-of-Its-Kind Consumer Guide to the Risks and Benefits of Volunteering for Clinical Trials." 2002. Retrieved September 1, 2004, from http://www.centerwatch.com/newsreleases/4-11-2002.html.

Chadwick, Gary. 1997. "Historical Perspective: Nuremberg, Tuskegee, and the Radiation Experiments." *Journal of the International Association of Physicians in AIDS Care* 3(1):27–28.

Chambliss, Daniel F. 1996. *Beyond Caring: Hospitals, Nurses, and the Social Organization of Ethics.* Chicago: University of Chicago Press.

Cherry, Brenda. 2005. "Drug Testing Goes Offshore." *Fortune* 8:66.

Cherry, Donald, David Woodwell, and Elizabeth Rechtsteiner. 2005. "National Ambulatory Medical Care Survey 2005 Summary." Division of Health Care Statistics, CDC. http://www.cdc.gov/nchs/data/ad/ad387.pdf.

Christakis, Nicholas. 1992. "Ethics Are Local: Engaging Cross-Cultural Variation in the Ethics for Clinical Research." *Social Science and Medicine* 35(9):1079–1091.

"Clinical Trials and Protection of Trial Subjects in Low-Income and Developing Countries." November 6, 2007. Final Report of the expert meeting, European Parliament and WEMOS. http://www.wemos.nl/Documents/report_expert_meeting_clinical_trials.pdf.

The Clinical Trials Business. 2003. Report B-171. Norwalk, CT: Business Communication Co.

ClinPage. 2007. "NEJM Indicts CROs." October 18. http://www.clinpage.com/article/nejm_indicts_cros/.

Cohen, Carl. 1978. "Medical Experimentation on Prisoners." *Perspectives in Biology and Medicine* 21:357–372.

Cohen, Jon. 2006. "The New World of Global Health." *Science* 311(5758):162–167.

Cohen, Lawrence. 1999. "Where It Hurts: Indian Material for an Ethics of Organ Transplantation. *Daedalus* 128(4):135–165.

Comaroff, John, and Jean Comaroff. 1992. "Medicine, Colonialism, and the Black Body." In *Ethnography and the Historical Imagination*, edited by Jean Comaroff and John Comaroff, 215–235. Boulder, CO: Westview Press.

———. 2006. *Law and Disorder in the Postcolony*. Chicago: University of Chicago Press.

"Comments on the Draft Health and Human Services Inspector General's Report: The Globalization of Clinical Trials." 2001. (OEI-01–00–00190) (HRG Publication #1591). *Public Citizen's Health Research Group*. July 5, 2001. Retrieved December 12, 2003, from http://www.citizen.org/publications/release.cfm?ID=7087&secID=1158&catID=126.

Cook-Deegan, Robert, and Tom Dedeurwaerdere. 2006. "The Science Commons in Life Science Research: Structure, Function, and Value of Access to Genetic Diversity." *International Social Science Journal* 58(188):299–317.

"CRO Industry at a Glance." 2007. *Association of Clinical Research Organizations*. Retrieved from http://www.acrohealth.org/industry-ataglance.php.

Crouch, Robert A., and John D. Arras. 1998. "AZT Trials and Tribulations." *Hastings Center Report* 28(6):26–34.

Daemmrich, Arthur A. 2004. *Pharmacopolitics: Drug Regulation in the United States and Germany*. Chapel Hill: University of North Carolina Press.

Das, Veena. 1995. "Suffering, Legitimacy, and Healing: The Bhopal Case." In *Critical Events: An Anthropological Perspective on Contemporary India*. Delhi: Oxford University Press.

———. 1999. "Public Good, Ethics, and Everyday Life: Beyond the Boundaries of Bioethics." *Daedalus* 128(4):99–134.

Das, Veena, and Ranendra Das. 2006. "Pharmaceuticals in Urban Ecologies: The Register of the Local." In *Global Pharmaceuticals: Ethics, Markets, Practices*, edited by Adriana Petryna, Andrew Lakoff, and Arthur Kleinman, 171–206. Durham, NC: Duke University Press.

Davidoff, Frank, Catherine D. DeAngelis, Jeffrey M. Drazen, M. Gary Nicholls, John Hoey, Liselotte Højgaard, Richard Horton, Sheldon Kotzin, Magne Nylenna, A. Overbeke, Harold C. Sox, Martin Weyden, and Michael S. Wilkes.

2001. "Sponsorship, Authorship and Accountability." *Journal of the American Medical Association* 286(10):1232–1234.

Davies, Norman. 2005. *Rising '44: The Battle for Warsaw.* New York: Penguin.

DeAngelis, C. D., J. M. Drazen, F. A. Frizelle, et al. 2004. "Clinical Trial Registration: A Statement from the International Committee of Medical Journal Editors." *Journal of the American Medical Association* 292:1363–1364.

———. 2005. "Is This Clinical Trial Fully Registered? A Statement from the International Committee of Medical Journal Editors." *Journal of the American Medical Association* 293:2927–2929.

Decision Memorandum. 2005. Memorandum from John K. Jenkins, M.D., and Paul J. Seligman, M.D., M.P.H. through Steven Galson, M.D., M.P.H. 5, 9 n.5 (April 6, 2005), http://www.fda.gov/cder/drug/infopage/COX2/NSAIDdecision Memo.pdf.

DelVecchio Good, Mary-Jo. 2001. "The Biotechnical Embrace." *Culture, Medicine and Psychiatry* 25(4):395–410.

de Vries, Raymond. 2004. "How Can We Help? From 'Sociology in' to 'Sociology of' Bioethics." *Journal of Law, Medicine, and Ethics* 32(2):279–293.

de Vries, Raymond, Adriana Petryna, Trudo Lemmens, Charles Bosk, and Jefferey Kahn. 2004. Research proposal manuscript: *The Global Market in Human Subjects: The Needs of Multinational Corporations and the Rights of National Citizens.*

de Zulueta, P. 2001. "Randomised Placebo-Controlled Trials and HIV-Infected Pregnant Women in Developing Countries: Ethical Imperialism or Unethical Exploitation?" *Bioethics* 15(4):289–311.

Dickersin, Kay, and Drummond Rennie. 2003. "Registering Clinical Trials." *Journal of the American Medical Association* 290(4):516.

DiMasi, Joseph A., Ronald W. Hansen, and Henry G. Grabowski. 2003. "The Price of Innovation: New Estimates of Drug Development Costs." *Journal of Health Economics* 22:151–185.

DNDWG [Drugs for Neglected Diseases Working Group]. 2001. "Fatal Imbalance: The Crisis in Research and Development for Drugs for Neglected Diseases." Geneva: MSF and DNDWG, downloadable at www.msf.org/source/access/2001/fatal/fatal.pdf.

Dodier, Nicolas. 2005. "Transnational Medicine in Public Arenas: AIDS Treatments in the South." *Culture, Medicine and Psychiatry* 29(3):285–307.

Donne, John. 2007. *Selected Poems.* New York: Penguin.

Dourada, M.I.C., M. A. Veras, D. Barreira, and A. M. de Brito. 2006. "AIDS Epidemic Trends after the Introduction of Antiretroviral Therapy in Brazil." *Revista de Saúde Pública* 40 (Suppl.):1–8.

Drinkard, Jim. 2005. "Drugmakers Go Furthest to Sway Congress." *USA Today*, April 25. Retrieved August 6, 2007, from http://www.usatoday.com/money/industries/health/drugs/2005-04-25-drug-lobby-cover_x.htm.

Dumit, Joseph. 2000. "When Explanations Rest: 'Good Enough' Brain Science and the New Biomental Disorders." In *Living and Working with the New Medical Technologies: Intersections of Inquiry*, edited by Margaret Lock, Alan Young, and Alberto Cambrosio, 209–233. Cambridge: Cambridge University Press.

————. Forthcoming. *Drugs for Life*. Durham, NC: Duke University Press.

Dunn, Elizabeth. 2004. *Privatizing Poland: Baby Food, Big Business, and the Remaking of Labor*. Ithaca: Cornell University Press.

Ecks, Stefan. 2005. "Pharmaceutical Citizenship: Antidepressant Marketing and the Promise of Demarginalization in India." *Anthropology & Medicine*. 12(3):239–254.

————. 2008. "Global Pharmaceutical Markets and Corporate Citizenship." *Biosocieties* 3:165–181.

Ejembi, C. L., E. P. Renne, and H. A. Adamu. 1998. "The Politics of the 1996 Cerebrospinal Meningitis Epidemic in Nigeria." *Africa: Journal of the International African Institute* 68(1):118–134.

Elias, Paulo Eduardo M., and Amelia Cohn. 2003. "Health Reform in Brazil: Lessons to Consider." *American Journal of Public Health* 93(1):44–48.

Elliott, Carl. 2007. "We'll Test It on Them." *American Prospect*, March 18. Available at http://www.prospect.org/cs/articles?article=well_test_it_on_them.

————. 2008. "Guinea Pigging." *New Yorker*, January 7.

Epstein, Helen. 2007. *The Invisible Cure: Africa, the West, and the Fight against AIDS*. New York: Farrar, Straus and Giroux.

Epstein, Steven. 1996. *Impure Science: AIDS, Activism, and the Politics of Knowledge*. Berkeley and Los Angeles: University of California Press.

————. 2007. *Inclusion: The Politics of Difference in Medical Research*. Chicago: University of Chicago Press.

Etkin, Nina. 1999. "The Rational Basis of 'Irrational' Drug Use: Pharmaceuticals in the Context of Development." In *Anthropology in Public Health: Bridging Differences in Culture and Society*, edited by Robert A. Hahn, 165–182. Oxford: Oxford University Press.

Faden, Ruth, Tom Beauchamp, and Nancy King. 1986. *The History and Theory of Informed Consent*. New York: Oxford University Press.

Farmer, Paul. 1999. *Infections and Inequalities: The Modern Plagues*. Berkeley and Los Angeles: University of California Press.

————. 2002. "Can Transnational Research Be Ethical in the Developing World?" *Lancet* 360(9342):1266–1302.

————. 2003. *Pathologies of Power: Health, Human Rights, and the New War on the Poor*. Berkeley and Los Angeles: University of California Press.

Finn, P. B. 2006. "The Negotiation and Development of a Clinical Trial Agreement." *Journal of Biolaw and Business* 9(2):21–27.

"Fiocruz culpa tradução incompleta por experimento com iscas humanas." *Folha Online*. Retrieved July 27, 2007, from http://www1.folha.uol.com.br/folha/cotidiano/ult95u116511.shtml.

Fischer, Michael M. J. 2001. "Ethnographic Critique and Technoscientific Narratives: The Old Mole, Ethical Plateaux, and the Governance of Emergent Biosocial Polities." *Culture, Medicine and Psychiatry* 25(4):355–393.

————. 2003. *Emergent Forms of Life and the Anthropological Voice*. Durham, NC: Duke University Press.

Fisher, Jill A. 2009. *Medical Research for Hire: The Political Economy of Pharmaceutical Clinical Trials*. New Brunswick, NJ: Rutgers University Press.

Fox, Renee. 1959. *Experiment Perilous: Physicians and Patients Facing the Unknown*. Glencoe, IL: Free Press.

Franklin, Sarah. 1995. "Science as Culture, Cultures of Science." *Annual Review of Anthropology* 24:163–185.

Friedman, Thomas. 2005. *The World Is Flat: A Brief History of the Twenty-first Century*. New York: Farrar, Straus and Giroux.

Frost, L., M. R. Reich, and T. Fujisaki. 2002. "A Partnership for Ivermectin: Social Worlds and Boundary Objects." In *Public-Private Partnerships for Public Health*, edited by M. R. Reich, 87–113. Cambridge: Harvard University Press.

"Future Developments for Gaucher Disease including Enzyme Replacement Therapy." 2002. Gaucher News. Retrieved from http://www.gaucher.org.uk/furthermarch2002.htm.

Galvão, Jane. 2002. "Access to Antiretroviral Drugs in Brazil." *Lancet* 360:1862–1865.

Garnier, J. P. 2005. Contribution at conference, Advancing Enterprise. February 4. Retrieved February 4, 2005, from http://www.hm-treasury.gov.uk/media/30C/C2/Dr_JP_Garnier.pdf.

Garrett, Laurie. 2007. "The Challenge of Global Health." *Foreign Affairs* 86 (1):14–38.

Geertz, Clifford. 1984 [2000]. "Anti Anti-Relativism." In *Available Light: Anthropological Reflections on Philosophical Topics*, 42–67. Princeton: Princeton University Press.

———. 2001. "Life among the Anthros." *New York Review of Books* 48(2):18–22.

Geissler, P. W., A. Kelly, B. Imoukhuede, and R. Pool. 2008. "'He is now like a brother, I can even give him some blood'—Relational Ethics and Material Exchanges in a Malaria Vaccine 'Trial Community' in the Gambia." *Social Science and Medicine* 67(5):696–707.

Geissler, P. W., and C. Molyneux, eds. In press. *African Trial Community: Ethnographies and Histories of Medical Research in Africa*. New York: Berghahn Publishers.

GFHR [Global Forum for Health Research]. 2004. *The 10/90 Report on Health Research 2003–2004*. Geneva: GFHR. Also at www.globalforumhealth.org/pages/index.asp.

Gilhooley, Margaret. 2007. "Vioxx's History and the Need for Better Procedures and Better Testing." *Seton Hall Law Review* 37:941–956.

Global Pharmaceuticals Sales Statistics. 2006. Retrieved August 5, 2007, from http://www.lesechos.fr/medias/2007/0323//300153931.pdf.

Godlee, Fiona. 2006. "An International Standard for Disclosure of Clinical Trial Information" (editorial). *British Medical Journal* 332:1107–1108.

Goodman, Jordan, Anthony McElligott, and Lara Marks. 2003. *Useful Bodies: Humans in the Service of Medical Science in the Twentieth Century*. Baltimore: Johns Hopkins University Press.

Goozner, Merrill. 2004. *The $800 Million Pill: The Truth behind the Cost of New Drugs*. Berkeley and Los Angeles: University of California Press.

Gorman, James. 2004. "The Altered Human Is Already Here." *New York Times*, April 6, F1.

Gostin, Lawrence. 2007. "Global Regulatory Strategies for Tobacco Control." *Journal of the American Medical Association* 298(17):2057–2058.

Graham, David. 2004. Statement of David J. Graham before the Senate Finance Committee Hearing, 108th Congress, "The FDA, Merck, and Vioxx: Putting Safety First." Washington, DC.

Greene, Jeremy. 2006. *Prescribing by Numbers: Drugs and the Definition of Disease.* Baltimore: Johns Hopkins University Press.

Greenhouse, Carol. 2005. "Hegemony and Hidden Transcripts: The Discursive Arts of Neoliberal Legitimation." *American Anthropologist* 107(3):356–368.

———. 2006. "Fieldwork on Law." *Annual Review of Law and Social Science* 2:187–210.

Greenslit, Nathan. 2005. "Depression and Consumption: Psychopharmaceuticals, Branding, and New Identity Practices." *Culture, Medicine and Psychiatry* 29(4):477–501.

"The Growing Power of the Fortune 500." 2006. *Working Life.* Labor Research Association. Downloaded August 5, 2007, from http://www.workinglife.org/wiki/.

Guidance for Industry: Information Program on Clinical Trials for Serious or Life-Threatening Diseases and Conditions. 2002. Washington, DC: U.S. Department of Health and Human Services, Food and Drug Administration, Center for Drug Evaluation and Research, Center for Biologics Evaluation and Research.

Guillemin, Jeanne. 1998. "Bioethics and the Coming of the Corporation to Medicine." In *Bioethics and Society,* edited by Raymond de Vries and Janardon Subedi, 60–77. Upper Saddle River, NJ: Prentice Hall.

Halperin, Daniel. 2008. "Putting a Plague in Perspective" (op-ed). *New York Times.* Available at http://www.nytimes.com/2008/01/01/opinion/01halperin.html.

Halpern, Sydney. 2001. "Constructing Moral Boundaries: Public Discourse on Human Experimentation in Twentieth-Century America." In *Bioethics in Social Context,* edited by Barry Hoffmaster, 69–89. Philadelphia: Temple University Press.

———. 2004. *Lesser Harms: The Morality of Risk in Medical Research.* Chicago: University of Chicago Press.

Hardon, Anita. 1987. "The Use of Modern Pharmaceuticals in a Filipino Village: Doctors' Prescription and Self-Medication." *Social Science and Medicine* 25(3):277–292.

Harkness, Jon M. 1996. "Research behind Bars: A History of Nontherapeutic Research on American Prisoners." Ph. D. diss., University of Wisconsin, Madison.

Harris, Gardiner. 2004a. "Drug Trial Finds Big Health Risks in 2nd Painkiller." *New York Times,* December 18, 2004.

———. 2004b. "New Study Links Pfizer's Bextra, Similar to Vioxx, to Heart Attacks." *New York Times,* November 10, 2004.

Hayden, Cori. 2007. "Taking as Giving: Bioscience, Exchange, and the Politics of Benefit-Sharing." *Social Studies of Science* 37(5):729–758.

Hawkins, J. S., and E. J. Emanuel. 2005. "Clarifying Confusions about Coercion." *Hastings Center Report* 35(5):16–19.

Health in the Americas. 1998. "Brazil." Pan American Health Organization. Retrieved from http://www.paho.org/English/HIA1998/Brazil.pdf.

Healy, David. 1999. *The Antidepressant Era.* Cambridge: Harvard University Press.

———. 2004. *Let Them Eat Prozac: The Unhealthy Relationship between the Pharmaceutical Industry and Depression.* New York: New York University Press.

———. 2006. "The New Medical Oikumene." In *Global Pharmaceuticals: Ethics, Markets, Practices,* edited by Adriana Petryna, Andrew Lakoff, and Arthur Kleinman, 61–85. Durham, NC: Duke University Press.

Heimer, Carol. 2008. "Expertise and Flexibility in Medicine and Law (What Happens When HIV Guidelines Are Hardened by Law)." Unpublished manuscript.

Heller, Jean. 2000. "Syphilis Victims in U.S. Study Went Untreated for Forty Years." In *Tuskegee's Truths: Rethinking the Tuskegee Syphilis Study,* edited by Susan M. Reverby, 116–119. Chapel Hill: University of North Carolina Press.

Hilts, Philip. 2004. *Protecting America's Health: The FDA, Business, and One Hundred Years of Regulation.* Chapel Hill: University of North Carolina Press.

Hirschman, Albert. 1970. *Exit, Voice, and Loyalty: Responses to Decline in Firms, Organizations, and States.* Cambridge: Harvard University Press.

———. 1980. "Morality and the Social Sciences: A Durable Tension." Acceptance Paper, the Frank E. Seidman Distinguished Award in Political Economy. Memphis, TN: P. K. Seidman Foundation, October.

Hoffman, Sharona. 2000. "Beneficial and Unusual Punishment: An Argument in Support of Prisoner Participation in Clinical Trials." *Indiana Law Review* 33:475–515.

Hornblum, Allen. 1991. *Acres of Skin: Human Experiments at Holmesburg Prison.* New York: Routledge.

Horrobin, David. 2002. "Effective Clinical Innovation: An Ethical Imperative." *Lancet* 359(9320):1857–1858.

Howell, J. D., and R. A. Hayward. 2003. "Writing Willowbrook, Reading Willowbrook: The Recounting of a Medical Experiment." In *Using Bodies: Humans in the Service of Medical Science in the Twentieth Century,* edited by J. Goodman, A. McElligott, and L. Marks, 190–213. Baltimore: Johns Hopkins University Press.

Huibers, Marcus J. H., Gijs Bleijenberg, Anna J.H.M. Beurskens, Ijmert Kant, J. André Knottnerus, Daniëlle A.W.M. van der Windt, Ellen Bazelmans, and Constant P. van Schayck. 2004. "An Alternative Trial Design to Overcome Validity and Recruitment Problems in Primary Care Research." *Family Practice* 21:213–218.

Humbert, Marc, Olivier Sitbon, and Gérald Simonneau. 2004. "Treatment of Pulmonary Arterial Hypertension." *New England Journal of Medicine* 351(14): 1425–1436.

Humpl, Tilman, Janette T. Reyes, Helen Holtby, Derek Stephens, and Ian Adatia. 2005. "Beneficial Effect of Oral Sildenafil Therapy on Childhood Pulmonary Arterial Hypertension." *Circulation* 111:3274–3280.

Hunt, Nancy. 1999. *A Colonial Lexicon: Of Birth Ritual, Medicalization, and Mobility in the Congo.* Durham, NC: Duke University Press.

Institute of Medicine. 2006. "The Future of Drug Safety: Promoting and Protecting the Health of the Public." Washington, DC: National Academies Press.

Iyalomhe, G. B., and P. A. Imomoh. 2007. "Ethics of Clinical Trials." *Nigerian Journal of Medicine* 16(4):301–306.

Jacob, Marie-Andrée, and Annelise Riles. 2007. "The New Bureaucracies of Virtue: Introduction." *PoLAR* 30(2):181–192.

Jain, Sarah Lochlann. 2006. *Injury: The Politics of Product Design and Safety Law in the United States.* Princeton: Princeton University Press.

Jasanoff, Sheila. 1998. *The Fifth Branch: Science Advisors as Policymakers.* Cambridge: Harvard University Press.

———. 2006. "Experiments without Borders: Biology in the Labs of Life." http://www.lse.ac.uk/collections/LSEPublicLecturesAndEvents/pdf/20060615_Jasanoff.pdf.

Jonas, Hans. 1969. "Philosophical Reflections on Human Experimentation." *Daedalus* 98:219–247.

Jones, James H. 1981 [1993]. *Bad Blood: The Tuskegee Syphilis Experiment.* New York: Free Press.

Jonsen, Albert R., and Jeff Stryker, eds. 1993. *The Social Impact of AIDS in the United States.* Washington, DC: National Academy of Sciences.

Juni, P., L. Nartey, S. Reichenbach, R. Sterchi, P. A. Dieppe, and M. Egger. 2004. "Risk of Cardiovascular Events and Rofecoxib: Cumulative Meta-Analysis." *Lancet* 364(9450):2021–2029.

Kahn, Jonathan. 2004. "How a Drug Becomes 'Ethnic': Law, Commerce, and the Production of Racial Categories in Medicine." *Yale Journal of Health Policy, Law, and Ethics* 4:1–46.

Kahn, J. P., A. C. Mastroianni, and J. Sugarman, eds. 1998. *Beyond Consent: Seeking Justice in Research.* New York: Oxford University Press.

Kalmbach, K. C., and Philip Lyons, Jr. 2003. "Ethical and Legal Standards for Research in Prisons." *Behavioral Sciences and the Law* 21(5):671–686.

Kassirer, Jerome P. 2004. *On the Take: How Medicine's Complicity with Big Business Can Endanger Your Health.* New York: Oxford University Press.

Kent, David M., Mkaya Mwamburi, et al. 2004. "Clinical Trials in Sub-Saharan Africa and Established Standards of Care: A Systematic Review of HIV, Tuberculosis, and Malaria Trials." *Journal of the American Medical Association* 292:237–242.

Kim, Jim Yong, Joia S. Mukherjee, Michael L. Rich, Kedar Mate, Jaime Bayona, and Mercedes Becerra. 2003. "From Multidrug-Resistant Tuberculosis to DOTS Expansion and Beyond: Making the Most of a Paradigm Shift." *Tuberculosis* 83(3):59–65.

Kimmelman, J. 2007. "Stable Ethics: Enrolling Non-treatment-refractory Volunteers in Novel Gene Transfer Trials." *Molecular Therapy* 15(11):1904–1906.

Klein, Naomi. 2007. *The Shock Doctrine: The Rise of Disaster Capitalism.* New York: Metropolitan Books.

Klein, Rudolf. 1980. "Models of Man and Models of Policy: Reflection on Exit,

Voice, and Loyalty Ten Years Later." *Milbank Memorial Fund Quarterly* 58(3): 416–429.

Kleinman, Arthur. 1981. *Patients and Healers in the Context of Culture.* Berkeley and Los Angeles: University of California Press.

———. 1999. "Moral Experience and Ethical Reflection: Can Ethnography Reconcile Them? A Quandary for 'The New Bioethics.'" *Daedalus* 128(4):69–99.

Konrad, Monica. 2007. "International Biodiplomacy and Global Ethical Forms: Relations of Critique between Public Anthropology and Science in Society." *Anthropological Quarterly* 80(2):325–353.

Krall, Hannah. 1996. *To Steal a March on God.* New York: Routledge.

Krimsky, Sheldon. 2003. *Science in the Private Interest.* Lanham, MD: Rowman & Littlefield.

Kuebler, Chris, Walter S. Nimmo, Joseph H. von Rickenbach, Dennis Gillings, Allan T. Morgan, Candace Kendle, and Paul S. Covington. 2002. "Ethics and Industry-Sponsored Research." *Canadian Medical Association Journal* 166 (5):580–581.

Kuo, Wen-Hua. 2005. "Japan and Taiwan in the Wake of Bio-Globalization: Drugs, Race and Standards." Ph.D. diss., Massachusetts Institute of Technology.

Laine, Christine, Richard Horton, Catherine D. DeAngelis, Jeffrey M. Drazen, Frank A. Frizelle, Fiona Godlee, Charlotte Haug, Paul C. Hébert, Sheldon Kotzin, Ana Marusic, Peush Sahni, Torben V. Schroeder, Harold C. Sox, Martin B. Van Der Weyden, and Freek W. A. Verheugt. 2007. "Clinical Trial Registration—Looking Back and Moving Ahead." *New England Journal of Medicine* 356(26):2734–2736.

Lakoff, Andrew. 2006a. "High Contact: Gifts and Surveillance in Argentina." In *Global Pharmaceuticals: Ethics, Markets, Practices,* edited by Adriana Petryna, Andrew Lakoff, and Arthur Kleinman, 111–136. Durham, NC: Duke University Press.

Lakoff, Andrew. 2006b. *Pharmaceutical Reason: Knowledge and Value in Global Psychiatry.* Cambridge: Cambridge University Press.

Lansbury, Peter. 2004. "An Innovative Drug Industry? Well, No." *Washington Post,* November 16, B02.

Lasagna, Louis. 1962. "Clinical Analysis of Medical Fads." *New York Times Magazine* 24(22):31–33.

———. 1977. "Prisoner Subjects and Drug Testing." *Federation Proceedings* 36(10):2349–2351.

Latour, Bruno. 1998. "Give Me a Laboratory and I Will Raise the World." In *The Science Studies Reader,* edited by Mario Biagioli, 258–275. New York: Routledge.

———. 2005. "From Realpolitik to Dingpolitik or How to Make Things Public." In *Making Things Public: Atmospheres of Democracy,* edited by Bruno Latour and Peter Weibel, 14–43. Cambridge, MA: MIT Press.

Lederer, Susan. 1997. *Subjected to Science: Human Experimentation in America before the Second World War.* Baltimore, MD: Johns Hopkins University Press.

Lederman, Rena. 2006. "Introduction: Anxious Borders between Work and Life in a Time of Bureaucratic Ethics Regulation." *American Ethnologist* 33(4):477–481.

Lemmens, Trudo, and Benjamin Freedman. 2000. "Ethics Review for Sale? Conflict of Interest and Commercial Research Review Boards." *Milbank Quarterly* 78:547–584.

Lemmens, Trudo, and Ron Bouchard. 2007. "Mandatory Clinical Trial Registration: Rebuilding Trust in Medical Research." In Global Forum for Health Research, *Global Forum Update on Research for Health*, vol. 4, *Equitable Access: Research Challenges for Health in Developing Countries.* London: Pro-Book Publishing.

Lerner, Barron H. 2007. "Subjects or Objects? Prisoners and Human Experimentation." *New England Journal of Medicine* 356(18):1806–1807.

Levine, C., R. Faden, C. Grady, D. Hammerschmidt, L. Eckenwiler, J. Sugarman; Consortium to Examine Clinical Research Ethics. 2004. "The Limitations of 'Vulnerability' as a Protection for Human Research Participants." *American Journal of Bioethics* 4(3):44–49.

Lewin, Tamar. 2001. "Families Sue Pfizer on Test of Antibiotic." *New York Times*, August 30, C1.

Lexchin, Joel. 2001. "Lifestyle Drugs: Issues for Debate." *Canadian Medical Association Journal* 164(10):1449–1451.

Lexchin, Joel, Lisa A. Bero, Benjamin Djulbegovic, and Otavio Clark. 2003. "Pharmaceutical Industry Sponsorship and Research Outcome and Quality: Systematic Review." *British Journal of Medicine* 326:1167–1170.

Light, Donald. 2008. "Reply to Dimasi, Hansen, and Grabowski." *Journal of Health Politics, Policy and Law* 33(2):325–327.

Light, Donald, and Rebecca Warburton. 2005. "Extraordinary Claims Require Extraordinary Evidence." *Journal of Health Economics* 24(5):1030–1033.

Lindenbaum, Shirley. 1978. *Kuru Sorcery: Disease and Danger in the New Guinea Highlands.* New York: McGraw-Hill.

Lippman, Abby. 2006. "The Inclusion of Women in Clinical Trials: Are We Asking the Right Questions?" March 2006. Toronto, ON: Women and Health Protection, http://www.whp-apsf.ca/en/documents/doc_index.html, downloaded November 7, 2007.

Lock, Margaret. 2001. *Twice Dead: Organ Transplants and the Reinvention of Death.* Berkeley and Los Angeles: University of California Press.

Love, James. "Health Care and Intellectual Property: The Orphan Drug Act." http://www.cptech.org/ip/healthorphan.

Lowy, Ilana. 2000. "Trustworthy Knowledge and Desperate Patients: Clinical Tests for New Drugs from Cancer to AIDS." In *Living and Working with the New Medical Technologies: Intersections of Inquiry*, edited by Margaret Lock, Alan Young, and Alberto Cambrosio, 49–82. Cambridge: Cambridge University Press.

Lurie, Peter, and Sidney M. Wolfe. 1998. "Unethical Trials of Interventions to Reduce Perinatal Transmission of the Human Immunodeficiency Virus in Developing Countries." *New England Journal of Medicine* 337(12):853–855.

———. 2000. "Letter to the National Bioethics Advisory Commission regarding Their Report on the Challenges of Conducting Research in Developing

Countries (HRG Publication #1545)." Accessed January 2007 at http://www
.citizen.org/publications/release.cfm?ID=6746.

Lustgarten, Abraham. 2005. "Drug Testing Goes Offshore." *Fortune*, August 8,
57–61.

Macklin, Ruth. 1999. *Against Relativism: Cultural Diversity and the Search for
Ethical Universals in Medicine.* Oxford: Oxford University Press.

———. 2004. *Double Standards in Medical Research in Developing Countries.*
Cambridge: Cambridge University Press.

Mansfield, Peter. 2006. "E-DRUG: Access to Essential Medicines as a Human
Right." Retrieved from http://www.essentialdrugs.org/edrug/archive/200607/
msg00078.php.

Marks, Harry. 1997. *The Progress of Experiment: Science and Therapeutic Reform
in the United States, 1900–1990.* Cambridge: Cambridge University Press.

———. 2000. "Where Do Ethics Come From? The Role of Disciplines and Institutions." Paper presented at the conference Ethical Issues in Clinical Trials,
University of Alabama at Birmingham, February 25.

———. 2002. Commentary. Third Annual W.H.R. Rivers Workshop, Global
Pharmaceuticals: Ethics, Markets, Practices. Harvard University, May 19–21.

———. 2008. "Making Risks Visible: The Science and Politics of Adverse Drug
Reactions." Unpublished manuscript.

Marks, Lara. 2001. *Sexual Chemistry: A History of the Contraceptive Pill.* New
Haven: Yale University Press.

Marshall, Patricia, and Barbara Koenig. 2004. "Accounting for Culture in a
Globalized Ethics." *Journal of Law, Medicine, and Ethics* 32(2):252–266.

Masters, B., and M. Kaufman. 2004. "Painful Withdrawal for Makers of Vioxx."
Washington Post, October 18, A01.

Mathews, Anna, and Barbara Martinez. 2004. "Warning Signs: E-Mails Suggest
Merck Knew Vioxx's Dangers at Early Stage—As Heart-Risk Evidence Rose,
Officials Played Hardball; Internal Message: 'Dodge!'—Company Says 'Out
of Context'." *Wall Street Journal*, November 1, A1.

McCabe, Christopher, Aki Tsuchiya, Karl Claxton, and James Raftery. 2006. "Drugs
for Exceptionally Rare Diseases: A Commentary on Hughes et al." University of
Sheffield, School of Health and Related Research, Discussion Paper Series.
Retrieved from http://www.shef.ac.uk/content/1/c6/01/87/47/0602FT.pdf.

Meadows, Michelle. 2002. "The FDA's Review Process: Ensuring Drugs Are Safe
and Effective." *FDA Consumer* 36 (July–August).

Medawar, Charles, and Anita Hardon. 2004. *Medicines out of Control? Antidepressants and the Conspiracy of Goodwill.* Amsterdam: Aksant Academic
Publishers.

Meinert, Curtis. 1988. "NIH Multicenter Investigator-Initiated Trials: An Endangered Species?" *Controlled Clinical Trials* 9:97–102.

———. 1995. "The Inclusion of Women in Clinical Trials." *Science* 269:795–796.

Meldrum, Marcia. 1994. "Departures from the Design: The Randomized Clinical Trial in Historical Context, 1946–1970." Ph.D. diss., State University of
New York at Stonybrook.

Melrose, Dianna. 1982. *Bitter Pills" Medicines and the Third World Poor*. Oxford: Oxfam.

Meng, Joyce. 2007. "Expanding Global Health Access: A Comparative Analysis of Pharmaceutical Corporate Social Responsibility Initiatives." Unpublished manuscript.

Merz, Jon F., David Magnus, Mildred K. Cho, and Arthur Caplan. 2002. "Protecting Subjects' Interests in Genetics Research." *American Journal of Human Genetics* 70(4):965–971.

Messeder, Ana Márcia. 2005. "Política Pública de Assistência Farmacêutica— Medicamentos de Dispensação em Caráter Excepcional." PowerPoint presentation. Departamento de assistência farmacêutica e insumos estratégicos/ SCTIE/MS. August 26.

Milne, C., and C. Paquette. 2004. "Meeting the Challenge of the Evolving R&D Paradigm: What Role for the CRO?" *American Pharmaceutical Outsourcing*. Available at www.americanpharmaceuticaloutsourcing.com.

Milosz, Czeslaw. 2004. *Second Space*. New York: Ecco.

Mirowski, Philip, and Esther-Mirjam Sent. 2007. "The Commercialization of Science and the Response of STS." In *Handbook of Science, Technology and Society Studies*, edited by E. Hackett, O. Amsterdamska, J. Wajcman, and Michael Lynch, 343–379. Cambridge, MA: MIT Press.

Mirowski, Philip, and Robert van Horn. 2005. "The Contract Research Organization and the Commercialization of Scientific Research." *Social Studies of Science* 35(4):503–548.

Misra, Kavita. 2000. "Productivity of Crises: Disease, Scientific Knowledge and State in India." *Economic and Political Weekly* 35(43–44):3885–3897.

Mitford, Jessica. 1973. "Experiments behind Bars: Doctors, Drug Companies, and Prisoners." *Atlantic Monthly* 23:64–73.

Moran, Mary. 2005. "A Breakthrough in R&D for Neglected Diseases: New Ways to Get the Drugs We Need." *PLoS Medicine* 2(9):302.

Moreno, Jonathan D. 1998. "Convenient and Captive Populations." In *Beyond Consent: Seeking Justice in Research*, edited by J. P. Kahn, A. C. Mastroianni, and J. Sugarman, 111–130. New York: Oxford University Press.

———. 2000. *Undue Risk: Secret State Experiments on Humans*. London: Routledge.

———. 2004. "Bioethics and the National Security State." *Journal of Law, Medicine, and Ethics* 32(2):198–208.

Moynihan, Ray, and Alan Cassels. 2005. *Selling Sickness: How the World's Biggest Pharmaceutical Companies Are Turning Us All into Patients*. New York: Nation Books.

Moynihan, Ray, Iona Heath, and David Henry. 2002. "Selling Sickness: The Pharmaceutical Industry and Disease Mongering." *British Medical Journal* 324:886–891.

Murthy, V. H., H. M. Krumholtz, and C. D. Gross. 2004. "Participation in Cancer Clinical Trials: Race-, Sex-, and Age-Based Disparities." *Journal of the American Medical Association* 291:2720–2726.

Nagengast, Carole, Michał Buchowski, and Edouard Conte, eds. 2001. *Poland beyond Communism: "Transition" in Critical Perspective.* Fribourg, Switzerland: University Press.

National Bioethics Advisory Commission. 2000. *Ethical and Policy Issues in International Research: Clinical Trials in Developing Countries.* Bethesda, MD: National Bioethics Advisory Commission.

Nguyen, Vinh-Kim. 2005. "Antiretroviral Globalism, Biopolitics, and Therapeutic Citizenship." In *Global Assemblages: Technology, Politics, and Ethics as Anthropological Problems,* edited by A. Ong and S. J. Collier, 124–144. Oxford: Blackwell.

Nichter, Mark. 2008. *Global Health: Why Cultural Perceptions, Social Representations, and Biopolitics Matter.* Tucson: University of Arizona Press.

Nichter, Mark, and Nancy Vuckovic. 1994. "Agenda for an Anthropology of Pharmaceutical Practice." *Social Science and Medicine* 39(11):1509–1525.

Notícias do CONASS. 2007. Retrieved July 7, 2007, from http://www.conass.org .br/.

OIG [Office of Inspector General, Department of Health and Human Services]. 2001. "The Globalization of Clinical Trials: A Growing Challenge in Protecting Human Subjects." Boston: Office of Evaluation and Inspections. Retrieved September 22, 2004, from http://oig.hhs.gov/organization/OIGmission .html.

———. 2007. "The Food and Drug Administration's Oversight of Clinical Trials." Retrieved September 30, 2007, from http://oig.hhs.gov/oei/reports/ oei-01-06-00160.pdf.

Okie, S. 2006. "Fighting HIV—Lessons from Brazil." *New England Journal of Medicine* 354(19):1977–1981.

Ong, Aihwa, and Stepen Collier, eds. 2005. *Global Assemblages: Technology, Politics, and Ethics as Anthropological Problems.* Malden, MA: Blackwell Publishing.

Ost, David. 2005. *The Defeat of Solidarity: Anger and Politics in Postcommunist Europe.* Ithaca: Cornell University Press.

Packard, Randall. 2007. *The Making of a Tropical Disease: A Short History of Malaria.* Baltimore: Johns Hopkins University Press.

Parexel. 2005. *Pharmaceutical R&D Statistical Sourcebook 2005/2006.* Waltham, MA: Parexel International.

———. 2008. *Bio/Pharmaceutical R&D Statistical Sourcebook 2007/2008.* Waltham, MA: Parexel International.

Peltzman, Sam. 1973. "An Evaluation of Consumer Protection Legislation: The 1962 Drug Amendments." *Journal of Political Economy* 81(5):1049–1091.

PEPFAR [The President's Emergency Plan for AIDS Relief]. 2006. Second Annual Report to Congress, U.S. Department of State. Released by the Office of the U.S. Global AIDS Coordinator February 8, 2006, 107. Available at http:// www.state.gov/s/gac/rl/61284.htm, downloaded November 2007.

Petryna, Adriana. 2002. *Life Exposed: Biological Citizens after Chernobyl.* Princeton: Princeton University Press.

———. 2005. "Ethical Variability: Drug Development and the Globalization of Clinical Trials." *American Ethnologist* 32(2):183–197.

————. 2007. "Clinical Trials Offshored: On Private Sector Science and Public Health." *BioSocieties* 2:21–40.

Petryna, Adriana, and Arthur Kleinman. 2006. "The Pharmaceutical Nexus: An Introduction." In *Global Pharmaceuticals: Ethics, Markets, Practices,* edited by Adriana Petryna, Andrew Lakoff, and Arthur Kleinman, 1–33. Durham, NC: Duke University Press.

Petryna, Adriana, Andrew Lakoff, and Arthur Kleinman, eds. 2006. *Global Pharmaceuticals: Ethics, Markets, Practices.* Durham, NC: Duke University Press.

Pharmbiosys Main Page. 2007. Retrieved March 3, 2007, from http://www.pharmbiosys.com.

The Physician Compensation Report. July 2003. Marblehead, MA: HCPro.

Piantados, Steven, and Jenet Wittes. 1993. "Politically Correct Clinical Trials." *Controlled Clinical Trials* 14:562–567.

Picon, Paulo. 2006. "Role of HTA in Evaluation and Regulation of New Technology in Emergent Economies: A Public Health Policy Perspective." PowerPoint presentation delivered at Health Technology Assessment International, Adelaide, July 5.

Picon, Paulo, K. M. Amaral, Guilherme Sander, and J. G. Reis. 2005. "Implementation of Brazilian Guidelines for Treatment of Hepatitis C: A Cost-Saving Intervention in the South of Brazil." *Italian Journal of Public Health* 2:259.

Picon, Paulo, and A. Beltrame. 2002. *Protocolos Clínicos e Diretrizes Terapêuticas: Medicamentos Excepcionais,* vol. 1. Porto Alegre: Grafica e Editora Pallotti.

Picon, Paulo, A. Beltrame, Andry Costa, Guilherme Sander, K. M. Amaral, and B. C. Krug. 2005. "Brazilian Guidelines for High-Cost Drugs: The Development of National Evidence-Based Public Health Policy." *Italian Journal of Public Health* 3:150–151.

Picon, Paulo, A. F. Costa, R. Kuchenbecker, and A. Beltrame. 2002. "Peginterferon alfa-2b plus Ribavirin for Chronic Hepatitis." *Lancet* 359(9302):263.

Picon, Paulo, Andry Costa, and Guilherme Sander. 2005. *Protocolos Clínicos UNIMED—POA.* Porto Alegre: Nova Prova.

Picon, Paulo, I. V. Schwartz, C. Krug, R. Guigliani, L.C.B. Lima, and J. G. Reis. 2005. "Maintaining Clinical Efficacy with Cost-Reduction in the Treatment of Gaucher Disease: An Example of Successful Experience in the South of Brazil." *Italian Journal of Public Health* 2:259.

PIH Guide to the Community-Based Treatment of HIV in Resource-Poor Settings. 2006. 2nd ed. Available at http://model.pih.org/.

Pine, Frances, and Haldis Haukanes, eds. 2005. *Social Security, Vulnerability and People at Risk: Gender and Generation in the Former Socialist Countries of Europe and Central Asia.* Centre for Women's and Gender Research Series, vol. 17. University of Bergen.

Pocock, Stuart. 2002. "The Pro's and Con's of Non-Inferiority (Equivalence) Trials." In *The Science of the Placebo: Toward an Interdisciplinary Research Agenda,* edited by Harry A. Guess, Arthur Kleinman, John W. Kusek, and Linda W. Engel, 236–248. London: BMJ Books.

Pogge, Thomas. 2006. "Harnessing the Power of Pharmaceutical Innovation." In *The Power of Pills: Social, Ethical, and Legal Issues in Drug Development,*

Marketing, and Pricing, edited by Jillian Claire Cohen, Patricia Illingworth, and Udo Schuklenk, 142–149. London: Pluto Press. Downloadable at http://www.colbio.org.mx/simposium_colbio/Thomas_Pogge.pdf.

———. 2007. "Could Globalization Be Good for World Health?" *Global Justice: Theory and Practice Rhetoric* 1:1–10.

Pollack, Andrew. 2007a. "Pricing Pills by the Results." *New York Times,* July 14, C1, C4.

———. 2007b. "Death in Gene Therapy Treatment Is Still Unexplained." *New York Times,* September 18, A22.

———. 2008. "Cutting Dosage of Costly Drug Spurs a Debate." *New York Times,* March 16, A1, A24.

Prakash, Gyan. 1999. *Another Reason: Science and the Imagination of Modern India.* Princeton: Princeton University Press.

PricewaterhouseCoopers. 2006. "Clinical Trials in Poland—Main Barriers to Industry Development." http://www.pwc.com/pl/eng/ins-sol/publ/2006/ph_badania_kliniczne.pdf.

Psaty, Bruce. 2004. Statement of Prof. Bruce Psaty before the Senate Finance Committee Hearing, 108th Congress, "The FDA, Merck, and Vioxx: Putting Safety First." Washington, DC.

Psaty, B. M., and C. D. Furberg. 2005. "COX-2 Inhibitors—Lessons in Drug Safety." *New England Journal of Medicine* 352:1135.

Psaty, Bruce M., and Richard A. Kronmal. 2008. "A Case Study Based on Documents from Rofecoxib Litigation." *Journal of the American Medical Association* 299(15):1813–1817.

Quintanilla, Ray. 2004. "Anger over Puerto Rico's Pill Test Lingers." *thebatt.com.* Texas A&M. Retrieved from http://www.thebatt.com/media/paper657/news/2004/04/12/.

Rabinow, Paul. 1996. *Essays on the Anthropology of Reason.* Princeton: Princeton University Press.

———. 2003. *Anthropos Today: Reflections on Modern Equipment.* Princeton: Princeton University Press.

Ramiah, Ilavenil, and Michael R. Reich. 2005. "Public-Private Partnerships and Antiretroviral Drugs for HIV/AIDS: Lessons from Botswana." *Health Affairs* 24(2):545–551.

Ramos, Joana D. 2004. "Gleevec Patient Assistance Program USA." Retrieved from http://ramoslink.info/pubs/GlivecPAP.pdf.

———. 2005. "New Definition of 'Patient Assistance Program' in Brazil." *Healthy Skepticism International News* 23:1.

Rapp, Rayna. 1999. *Testing Women, Testing the Fetus: The Social Impact of Amniocentesis in America.* New York: Routledge.

Rasmussen, Nicholas. 2005. "Drugs and Globalisation." *Metascience* 14:73–77.

Redfield, Peter. 2006. "A Less Modest Witness: Collective Advocacy and Motivated Truth in a Medical Humanitarian Movement." *American Ethnologist* (33)1:3–26.

RedFearn, Suz. 2008. "We're Not Sweatshops: ACRO Responds to NEJM." http://www.clinpage.com/article/acro_responds_to_nejm/.

Reich, Michael R., ed. 2002. *Public-Private Partnerships for Public Health.* Cambridge, MA: Harvard Center for Population and Development Studies.

Relman, Arnold, and Marcia Angell. 2002. "How the Drug Industry Distorts Medicine and Politics: America's Other Drug Problem." *New Republic,* December 16, 27–41.

Rettig, Richard. 2000. "The Industrialization of Clinical Research." *Health Affairs* 19(2):129–146.

Reverby, Susan, ed. 2000. *Tuskegee's Truths: Rethinking the Tuskegee Syphilis Study.* Chapel Hill: University of North Carolina Press.

Rheinberger, Hans-Jorg. 1995. "From Experimental Systems to Cultures of Experimentation." In *Concepts, Theories, and Rationality in the Biological Sciences,* edited by G. Wolters, J. Lennox, and P. McLaughlin. Pittsburgh, PA: University of Pittsburgh Press.

Riles, Annelise. 2000. *The Network Inside Out.* Ann Arbor: University of Michigan Press.

———. 2004. "The Network Inside Out." In *The Anthropology of Development and Globalization: From Classical Political Economy to Contemporary Neoliberalism,* edited by Marc Edelman and Angelique Haugerud, 262–269. Hoboken, NJ: Wiley-Blackwell.

———. 2005. "Skepticism, Intimacy and the Ethnographic Subject: Human Rights as Legal Knowledge." *American Anthropologist,* December 2005. Available at SSRN: http://ssrn.com/abstract=742569.

———. 2006. "Anthropology, Human Rights, and Legal Knowledge: Culture in the Iron Cage." *American Anthropologist* 108(1):52–65.

Ringelblum, Emanuel. 1974. *Notes from the Warsaw Ghetto.* New York: Schocken.

Rivkin-Fish, Michele. 2005. *Women's Health in Post-Soviet Russia: The Politics of Intervention.* Bloomington: Indiana University Press.

Roitman, Janet. 2004. *Fiscal Disobedience: An Anthropology of Economic Regulation in Central Africa.* Princeton: Princeton: University Press.

Rosenberg, Roger N. 2003. "Translating Biomedical Research to the Bedside: A National Crisis and a Call to Action" (editorial). *Journal of the American Medical Association* 289(10):1305–1306.

Rothman, David. 1991. *Strangers at the Bedside: A History of How Law and Bioethics Transformed Medical Decision Making.* New York: Basic Books.

———. 2000. "The Shame of Medical Research." *New York Review of Books* 47(19):60–64.

Rothman, Sheila, and David Rothman. 2005. *The Willowbrook Wars.* New York: Aldine.

Sachs, Jeffrey. 2006. *The End of Poverty: Economic Possibilities for Our Time.* New York: Penguin.

Sackett, David, and Andrew Oxman. 2003. "HARLOT plc: An Amalgamation of the World's Two Oldest Professions." *British Medical Journal* 327:1442–1445.

Salter, Brian, Melinda Cooper, and Amanda Dickins. 2006. "China and the Global Stem Cell Bioeconomy: An Emerging Political Strategy?" *Regenerative Medicine* 1(5):671–683.

Samsky, Ari. 2008. "Pharmaceutical Philanthropy: An Anthropological Study of Practices and Values Shaping Drug Donations." Ph.D. diss., Princeton University.

Sander, Guilherme, Paulo Picon, F. D. Fuchs, A. Beltrame, and R. R. De Souza. 2003. "PEG-Interferon versus Conventional Interferon and Liver Fibrosis: Do We Have Evidence of Superiority?" *Gastroenterology* 124(2):584.

Sassen, Saskia. 2006. *Territory, Authority, Rights: From Medieval to Global Assemblages.* Princeton: Princeton University Press.

Scheper-Hughes, Nancy. 1992. *Death without Weeping: The Violence of Everyday Life in Brazil.* Berkeley and Los Angeles: University of California Press.

———. 2004. "Parts Unknown: Undercover Ethnography of the Organs-Trafficking Underworld." *Ethnography* 5(1):29–74.

Schmidt, Maria Inês, and Bruce B. Duncan. 2004. "Academic Medicine as a Resource for Global Health: The Case of Brazil." *British Medical Journal* 329: 753–754.

Schmit, Julie. 2005. "Costs, Regulations Move More Drug Tests Outside USA." *USA Today*, May 16.

Schuklenk, Udo, and R. Ashcroft. 2000. "International Research Ethics." *Bioethics* 14(2):158–172.

"Seminário discute ações judiciais sobre medicamentos excepcionais." 2005. *Agência Minas.* Retrieved from http://www.agenciaminas.mg.gov.br/detalhe_noticia.php?cod_noticia=5812.

Sewankambo, Nelson. 2004a. "Academic Medicine Needs a Global Agenda." *British Medical Journal* 329:751–752.

———. 2004b. "Academic Medicine and Global Health Responsibilities." *British Medical Journal* 329:752–753.

Shah, Sonia. 2007. *Body Hunters: How the Drug Industry Tests Its Products on the World's Poorest Patients.* New York: The New Press.

Shuchman, Miriam. 2007. Commercializing Clinical Trials—Risks and Benefits of the CRO Boom." *New England Journal of Medicine* 357(14):1365–1368.

Sieder, Rachel, Line Schjolden, and Alan Angell, eds. 2005. *The Judicialization of Politics in Latin America.* New York: Palgrave Macmillan.

Silverman, M., P. R. Lee, and M. Lydecker. 1982. *Prescriptions for Death: The Drugging of the Third World.* Berkeley and Los Angeles: University of California Press.

Sim, Ida, and Don E. Detmer. 2005. "Beyond Trial Registration: A Global Trial Bank for Clinical Trial Reporting." *PLoS Medicine* 2(11):1090–1092.

Simon, Gregory. 2006. "The Antidepressant Quandary—Considering Suicide Risk When Treating Adolescent Depression." *New England Journal of Medicine* 355(26):2722–2723.

Sinackevich, Nick, and Jean-Pierre Tassignon. 2004. "Speeding the Critical Path." *Applied Clinical Trials* 13(1):42–48.

Sivaramakrishnan, K. 2005. Introduction to "Moral Economies, State Spaces, and Categorical Violence." *American Anthropologist* 107(3):321–330.

Smith, Jane. 1990. *Patenting the Sun: Polio and the Salk Vaccine.* New York: William Morrow.

Steinbrook, Robert. 2005. "Gag Clauses in Clinical-Trial Agreements." *New England Journal of Medicine* 352(21):2160–2162.

Stephens, Trent D., and Rock Brynner. 2001. *Dark Remedy: The Impact of Thalidomide and Its Revival as a Vital Medicine.* Cambridge, MA: Perseus Publishing.

Stiglitz, Joseph. 2002. *Globalization and Its Discontents.* W. W. Norton & Company.

Strathern, Marilyn. 1992. *After Nature: English Kinship in the Late Twentieth Century.* Cambridge: Cambridge University Press.

Sunder Rajan, Kaushik. 2005. "Subjects of Speculation: Emergent Life Sciences and Market Logics in the United States and India." *American Anthropologist* 107(1):19–30.

———. 2006. *Biocapital: The Constitution of Postgenomic Life.* Durham, NC: Duke University Press.

———. 2007. "Experimental Values." *New Left Review* 45(May–June):67–88.

Sung, Nancy S., William F. Crowley Jr., Myron Genel, Patricia Salber, Lewis Sandy, Louis M. Sherwood, Stephen B. Johnson, Veronica Catanese, Hugh Tilson, Kenneth Getz, Elaine L. Larson, David Scheinberg, E. Albert Reece, Harold Slavkin, Adrian Dobs, Jack Grebb, Rick A. Martinez, Allan Korn, and David Rimoin. 2003. "Central Challenges Facing the National Clinical Research Enterprise." *Journal of the American Medical Association* 289:1278–1287.

Temple, Robert. 2002. "Placebo-Controlled Trials and Active Controlled Trials: Ethics and Inference." In *The Science of the Placebo: Toward an Interdisciplinary Research Agenda,* edited by Harry A. Guess, Arthur Kleinman, John W. Kusek, and Linda W. Engel, 209–227. London: BMJ Books.

Thiers, Fabio, Anthony Sinskey, and Ernst Berndt. 2007. "Trends in the Globalization of Clinical Trials." *Nature Reviews Drug Discovery* 7:13–14.

Timimi, Sami. 2007. Review of *Global Pharmaceuticals: Ethics, Markets, Practices. British Journal of Psychiatry* 190:367.

Timmermans, Stefan, and Marc Berg. 2003. *The Gold Standard: The Challenge of Evidence-Based Medicine.* Philadelphia: Temple University Press.

Topol, Eric J. 2004. "Failing the Public Health—Rofecoxib, Merck, and the FDA." *New England Journal of Medicine* 351:1707.

———. 2005. "Arthritis Medicines and Cardiovascular Events—'House of Coxibs.'" *Journal of the American Medical Association* 293(3):366–368.

Topol, Eric, and David Blumenthal. 2005. "Physicians and the Investment Industry." *Journal of the American Medical Association* 294(15):1897–1898.

Toulmin, Stephen. 1982. "How Medicine Saved the Life of Ethics." *Perspectives in Biology and Medicine* 25(4):736–750.

———. 1987. "National Commission on Human Experimentation: Procedures and Outcomes." In *Scientific Controversies: Case Studies in the Resolution and Closure of Disputes in Science and Technology,* edited by H. Tristram Engelhardt Jr. and Arthur L. Caplan, 599–615. Cambridge: Cambridge University Press.

Town Topics. 2004. Obituary of G. Hein Besselaar. Retrieved from http://www.towntopics.com/mar2404/obits.html.

"Treatment of Lysosomal Storage Disorders" (editorial). 2003. *British Medical Journal* 327:462–463.

"Trials of War Criminals before the Nuremberg Military Tribunals under Control Council Law No. 10." 1949. *Nuremberg Code.* No. 10, 181–182. Washington DC: U.S. Government Printing Office.

Tsing, Anna Lowenhaupt. 2004. *Friction: An Ethnography of Global Connection.* Princeton: Princeton University Press,

U.S. Department of Health and Human Services, Food and Drug Administration. 1998. "Investigational New Drug Applications and New Drug Applications, Final Rule." *Federal Register* 63(8):6854–6862.

U.S. Department of Health and Human Services, Food and Drug Administration, et al. 2005. Guidance for Industry Collection of Race and Ethnicity Data in Clinical Trials. Available at http://www.fda.gov/CbER/gdlns/racethclin.htm.

U.S. Food and Drug Administration. 2001. "International Conference on Harmonisation: Choice of Control Group and Related Issues in Clinical Trials." *Federal Register* 66:24390–24391.

———. 2002. "The FDA's Drug Review Process: Ensuring Drugs Are Safe and Effective." Retrieved May 12, 2006, from http://www.fda.gov/fdac/features/2002/402_drug.html.

———. 2007. "FDA's Critical Path Initiative—Science Enhancing the Health and Well-Being of All Americans." Retrieved March 2007, from http://www.fda.gov/oc/initiatives/criticalpath/initiative.html.

U.S. Food and Drug Administration, Office of Orphan Products Development. "OOPD Program Overview." Retrieved from http://www.fda.gov/orphan/progovw.htm.

U.S. National Institutes of Health. 2006. "Glossary of Clinical Trial Terms." National Library of Medicine. Retrieved August 7, 2007, from http://clinicaltrials.gov/ct/info/glossary.

———. 2007. "An Introduction to Clinical Trials." National Library of Medicine. Retrieved August 7, 2007, from http://clinicaltrials.gov/ct/info/whatis#phases.

"Uso de cobaias humanas no Amapá causa horror, diz senador da Folha." 2006. Retrieved July 27, 2007, from http://www1.folha.uol.com.br/folha/ciencia/ult306u14130.shtml.

Van der Geest, Sjaak, and Susan Reynolds Whyte, eds. 1988. *The Context of Medicines in Developing Countries: Studies in Pharmaceutical Anthropology.* Boston: Kluwer Academic Publishers.

Van der Geest, Sjaak, Susan Reynolds Whyte, and Anita Hardon. 1996. "The Anthropology of Pharmaceuticals: A Biographical Approach." *Annual Review of Anthropology* 25:153–178.

Varmus, Harold, and David Satcher. 1996. "Ethical Complexities of Conducting Research in Developing Countries." *New England Journal of Medicine* 337 (14):1003–1005.

Vastag, Brian. 2000. "Helsinki Discord? A Controversial Declaration." *Journal of the American Medical Association* 284(23):2983–2985.

Vaughan, Megan. 1992. *Curing Their Ills: Colonial Power and African Illness.* Stanford: Stanford University Press.

Vitoria, Cesar G., Jean-Pierre Habicht, and Jennifer Bryce. 2004. "Evidence-

Based Public Health: Moving beyond Randomized Trials." *American Journal of Public Health* 94(3):400–405.

Wardell, William, and Louis Lasagna. 1975. *Regulation and Drug Development.* Washington, DC: American Enterprise Institute for Public Policy Research.

Wedel, Janine. 1992. *The Unplanned Society: Poland during and after Communism.* New York: Columbia University Press.

Wendler, David, Kington Raynard, Jennifer Madans, Gretchen Van Wye, Heidi Christ-Schmidt, Laura A. Pratt, Otis W. Brawley, Cary P. Gross, and Ezekiel Emanuel. 2006. "Are Racial and Ethnic Minorities Less Willing to Participate in Health Research?" *PLoS Medicine* 3(2):0201–0210.

Wertheimer, Alan. 2006. *Coercion.* Princeton: Princeton University Press.

Whitmarsh, Ian. 2008. *Biomedical Ambiguity: Race, Asthma, and the Contested Meaning of Genetic Research in the Caribbean.* Ithaca: Cornell University Press.

Whyte, Susan Reynolds, Michael A. Whyte, Lotte Meinert, and Betty Kyaddondo. 2006. "Treating AIDS: Dilemmas of Unequal Access in Uganda." In *Global Pharmaceuticals: Ethics, Markets, Practices,* edited by Adriana Petryna, Andrew Lakoff, and Arthur Kleinman, 240–263. Durham, NC: Duke University Press.

Winter, Jane, and Jane Baguley. 2006. *Outsourcing Clinical Development: Strategies for Working with CROs and Other Partners.* Aldershot, UK: Ashgate Publishing.

Wood, Alastair J. J. 2006. "A Proposal for Radical Changes in the Drug-Approval Process." *New England Journal of Medicine* 355:618, 619, 622.

Woolf, Steven H., and Robert E. Johnson. 2005. "The Break-Even Point: When Medical Advances Are Less Important Than Improving the Fidelity with Which They Are Delivered." *Annals of Family Medicine* 3:545–552.

World Medical Association. 2000. "Declaration of Helsinki. Ethical Principles for Medical Research involving Human Subjects." *Journal of the American Medical Association* 284(23):3043–3045.

Young, Iris. 2004. "Responsibility and Historic Injustice." Paper presented at the School of Social Science Thursday Seminar, Institute for Advanced Study, Princeton, New Jersey, February 19.

Zarin, Deborah A., Nicholas C. Ide, Tony Tse, William R. Harlan, Joyce C. West, and Donald A. B. Lindberg. 2007. "Issues in the Registration of Clinical Trials." *Journal of the American Medical Association* 297(19):2112–2120.

Zarin, D. A., and A. Keselman. 2007. "Registering a Clinical Trial in Clinical Trials.gov." *Chest* 131(3):909–912.

INDEX